The Mediterranean Diet

Wine, Pasta, Olive Oil, and
a Long, Healthy Life

Also by Malcolm McConnell

FICTION

Matata
Clinton Is Assigned
Just Causes

NONFICTION

First Crossing *(with Carol McConnell)*
Stepping Over
Into the Mouth of the Cat
Middle Sea Autumn *(with Carol McConnell)*
The Essence of Fiction
Incident at Big Sky *(with Johnny France)*
Challenger: A Major Malfunction

The Mediterranean
D I E T

Wine, Pasta, Olive Oil,
and a Long, Healthy
Life

by Carol and Malcolm McConnell

W. W. Norton & Company *New York London*

Published simultaneously in Canada by Penguin Books Canada Ltd.,
2801 John Street, Markham, Ontario L3R 1B4.
Printed in the United States of America.

The text of this book is composed in Avanta, with
display type set in Caslon Bold Condensed and Century Old Style Bold
Composition and manufacturing by The Haddon Craftsmen, Inc.
Book design by Margaret M. Wagner.

First Edition

Library of Congress Cataloging-in-Publication Data

McConnell, Carol.
The Mediterranean diet.

Includes index.
1. Nutrition. 2. Longevity. 3. Diet—Mediterranean
Region. 4. Cookery, Mediterranean. I. McConnell,
Malcolm. II. Title.
RA784.M39 1987   613.2' 6   86–23840

ISBN 0-393-02438-5

W. W. Norton & Company, Inc., 500 Fifth Avenue, New York, N. Y. 10110
W. W. Norton & Company Ltd., 37 Great Russell Street, London WC1B 3NU

1 2 3 4 5 6 7 8 9 0

To the people of Lindos,
who taught us about
Mediterranean food.

Contents

Part III: Stress, Leisure, and Food

Acknowledgments

Our work is based on professional medical and nutritional research, not on the speculation of amateurs. We could not have written the book without the generous assistance of many people and organizations.

The World Health Organization provided us with a large and detailed statistical matrix in which we could compare the health patterns of the people of the Mediterranean Basin with the patterns of people from other parts of the the world. The WHO's extensive medical library in Geneva contained scores of research studies that we used to document our findings. We also used the National Medical Library at the National Institutes of Health in Bethesda, Maryland.

In Greece, Drs. Christos Aravanis, Paul Ioannidis, and Antonia Trichopoulou shared with us their impressive research.

Wine Institute and the Winegrowers of California made available to us their libraries of international research and cross-cultural studies on wine.

Dr. Scott Grundy of the University of Texas Health Science Center in Dallas generously shared his important recent findings on olive oil.

The International Olive Oil Council, which administers the International Olive Oil Agreement (IOOC), helped us a great deal with our sections on olive oil. We wish to thank its executive secretariat and the members of the IOOC: Algeria, Arab Republic of Egypt, the European Economic Community (Belgium, Britain, Denmark, France, Federal Republic of Germany, Greece, Ireland, Italy, Luxembourg, the Netherlands, Portugal, Spain), Socialist People's Libyan Arab Jamahiriya, Morocco, Tunisia, Turkey, and Yugoslavia.

Finally, the Research Department of Reader's Digest rigorously scrutinized our basic findings, which were incorporated into a *Digest* article published in September 1986. We thank them for their independent judgment and professionalism.

Introduction:
The Diet-Book "Midway"

Webster's defines the word *midway* as that part of a fair or an exposition where we may find "curiosities and games of chance," among other amusements. The midway's attractions are staffed by barkers, who, the dictionary tells us, are people employing "voluble glib speech or patter . . . to attract a crowd."

Let's substitute the image of a carnival midway, noisy with the chants of the barkers, for the diet-and-health section of a shopping-mall bookstore. Instead of Toby the Two-Headed Dog and the Wheel of Fortune, the books on the shelves invite us to step right up and discover an amazing (and often confusingly contradictory) variety of nutritional secrets. If only we follow the authors' persuasive patter, the dust jackets proclaim, we can remain fit and trim for life, avoid serious illness, gain astounding physical and emotional energy, recharge the power of our immune system, revitalize our sex lives, and, in general, protect ourselves from the slings and arrows of outrageous fortune. Not bad for $17.95.

Many of these books are specifically targeted for those millions of Americans who want to lose weight. Others promise general good health through radical shifts in eating habits that emphasize one form of food—raw fruit, for example—over all others. The authors sometimes offer arcane rationales for their nontraditional diets. Only they, it is suggested, understand the "true" mysteries of human metabolism. Perhaps their spiel comes in the form of testimonials from those star athletes whom they have restored to greatness through daily doses of sweet potatoes and bean sprouts. One book tells us never to eat meat; another admonishes us to eat meat only after noon; and so forth.

These books have become so popular that the *New York Times Book Review* was recently obliged to add an "Advice, How-to and Miscellaneous" section to its weekly list of best sellers. And salvation-through-diet books regularly share this section with titles that teach us how to manage our own divorce cases and rebuild the backyard deck. But such radical nutrition books are increasingly coming under attack from mainstream health professionals. These diet panaceas, doctors charge, often are wrong and sometimes dangerous.

Why, therefore, do we have the temerity to write yet another book of nutritional secrets that not only promises to protect you from life's most dread diseases and to make you feel better, but offers tasty, satisfying food as well? Are we not donning the barker's gaudy blazer and reaching for the megaphone when we suggest that you step right up and learn all about the life-saving benefits of traditional Mediterranean food?

Be aware at the outset that we are *not* promising you the moon and stars. We do not claim any astounding mystical insights into the vital diet-disease relationship. Our book is not based on controversial theories or a few case histories of champion tennis players or NFL quarterbacks. Throughout this book, you will see the phrases "common sense" and "moderation." The experts we cite are mainstream physicians and nutritionists from the World Health Organization (WHO), the National Institutes of Health, the American Heart Association, and the country's leading medical research facilities. In addition, we do not rely on vague claims distilled from anonymous "recent research." The reader will notice in our extensive Notes section that we substantiate all of our major conclusions with verifiable sources. And these sources are often the most authoritative and widely respected scientific journals in the world: the *Journal of the American Medical Association,* the *New England Journal of Medicine,* the *Lancet, Circulation,* and the *American Journal of Clinical Nutrition.* Finally, we draw upon a wide body of international research findings, which, unfortunately, until recently have often been overlooked by American nutritional experts.

Further, since the diet we're suggesting will not necessarily help you to lose weight, this is not a "diet" book in that regard. Weight reduction is *not* one of our primary goals; overall good health and well-being are. As far as we've been able to determine, after interviewing some of the world's nutritional experts, there is only one proven method for healthy adults to lose weight: eat fewer calories, and exercise more. And we certainly do suggest that you consider this method.

If he or she is lucky, everybody reading these words will grow old and feeble one day and will die. No "midway diet" guru can change that. But we do suggest that people can adopt a pattern of nutrition that will offer dramatic, increased protection from the two leading killers in the industrialized world: cardiovascular disease and cancer.

We began our project without a thesis or theory but with a long-term observation. Having lived in various parts of the Mediterranean Basin—Morocco, Italy, and Greece—during the past twenty years, we noticed that the people of this region who follow a traditional diet based on the "Mediterranean triad" of wheat, olives, and grapes appear amazingly healthy, despite their visible poverty and often primitive living conditions.[1]

Like most journalists, we filed away this seemingly trivial piece of information for possible future use. But we also realized that what we were observing could be isolated phenomena or that we were misinterpreting what we saw. Perhaps the people in Moroccan towns like Chechaouèn and Souk-el-Arba-du-Rharb or on small Greek islands such as Khálki and Kárpathos simply represented tough adult survivors, the living victors in a cruel natural-selection struggle that decimated the weaker individuals in infancy and childhood. Perhaps they owed their apparent health to good luck and good genes, not to the way they lived and ate. The suspicion lingered, however, that the traditional Mediterranean villager lived a healthy life that included a uniquely beneficial diet.

Then, recently, we had the chance to transform our observation into a thesis—and to prove it—when Reader's Digest funded our research on the article "Ancient Secrets of Modern Nutrition." What we discovered was so dramatic that we felt compelled to continue our research and expand the article into a full-length book.

During the course of this research, it has become clear that for millions of people the unique combination of foods in the traditional Mediterranean diet has dramatically reduced the incidence of heart disease and cancer. Armed with this information and encouraged by the international experts we consulted during our research, we decided to erect our own literary side show on the crowded diet-book "midway." We hope, however, that our effort is an exercise in common sense and not a flimflam act.

According to the World Health Organization's Expert Committee on Cardiovascular Disease, which studied the prevention of coronary heart disease, the people of the Mediterranean Basin (and parts of the Orient) "have low coronary heart disease (CHD) rates, are well nourished, show no excess of *non*cardiovascular disease mortality and have good life expectancy at all ages."[2]

In other words, they are protected from much of the heart disease and cancer that strikes down millions of northern Europeans and Americans each year. The head of the WHO's European Nutritional Division, Dr. Elizabet Helsing, calls cancer and CHD the "diseases of affluence" and blames their increased incidence directly on the high-animal-fat, high-calorie, low-vegetable, and low-fiber diets common today in many industrialized nations.[3]

A large proportion of Mediterraneans live long, healthy lives, relatively free of heart disease and cancer, because their traditional poverty has *forced* them to follow a moderate diet. In addition, this diet includes certain key components that have only recently been shown to offer great health benefits.[4]

What the understated bureaucratic prose of the WHO's Expert Committee does not reveal, however, is that the food of these healthy Mediterraneans is not just good for you, it offers a delicious alternative to the immoderately unhealthy diet that became the norm in this century.

PART I

Health, Diet, and the Mediterranean Triad

C H A P T E R 1

The Mediterranean Triad

In *The Ancient World,* the American classicist Paul MacKendrick introduces the term "Mediterranean triad" to describe the region's traditional agricultural underpinnings: wheat, olives, and grapes and wine.[1] Classical society ultimately depended on agriculture—on farmers and the food they grew; in turn, ancient farmers depended on climate, which controlled the annual cycles of rain and drought, heat and cold.

And the climate of the Mediterranean has remained comparatively stable since classical times: hot, dry summers and mild, rainy winters. This characteristic weather pattern shaped the region's main crops. The typical short-stalked durum wheat could ripen quickly in the warm, rainy spring and be harvested before the five-month summer drought burned the crop and baked the soil brick-hard. Olive trees, with their thick, gnarled trunks and deep taproots, could survive the dry summer but could not withstand prolonged freezing weather. Indeed, one could define the "Mediterranean" world as the region in which the olive grows.[2] And for almost eight thousand years, vineyards have flourished in the same soil and climate as the olive.

Given the relatively poor soil and harsh, rainless summer of the Mediterranean Basin, we may speculate that fast-growing spring wheat and drought-resistant olives and grapes were among the few staple crops that could have survived so well and have supported so many diverse Mediterranean civilizations for so many thousands of years.[3] One should also bear in mind that the area's poor soil led to erosion on a massive scale, which, in turn, produced a generally undependable water table. The Romans, in an attempt to correct this situation, built thousands of miles of aqueducts that brought water from the mountains to the coastal cities.

Even today, many Mediterranean villages do not have a dependable year-round water supply; villagers must supplement the water from the town well with water from household cisterns. In antiquity, the staple foods of the Mediterranean, therefore, had to be grown without the benefit of regular annual rainfall, and farmers had to be able to process these staple crops into nutritious food that would last throughout the year without refrigeration and would provide a balanced diet. In this regard, the triad of wheat, olives, and grapes was ideal.

Wheat can be stored as raw grain for years or processed into flour or pasta. And even in a bad year, one grain crop can be wrested from the earth and laid away as whole-grain flour, semolina, or pasta.

Olives can be easily preserved as either green or ripe fruit and can provide palatable, high-quality nutrition year-round. The oil obtained from pressing the olives can be kept nearly indefinitely. Olive oil represents a cash crop that has, with wine, been a major source of income for Mediterranean farmers.

And the grape can serve many needs: as fresh fruit, as dried fruit (currants and raisins), and especially as wine, the ubiquitous gift of Bacchus found across the Mediterranean world. Since the dawn of history, wine has played a vital role in Mediterranean commerce and culture. Wine, like olive oil, is the preserved essence of the soil. Moderate consumption of wine with meals can be found in almost every Mediterranean culture, including the Muslim cultures of Turkey and the North African Maghreb (Morocco, Algeria, Tunisia, and, until recently, Libya). Wine is as natural a part of the triad as are wheat and olives. As we shall see, the health benefits of wine are widespread and varied.

Since Biblical times, Mediterraneans have based their diet on this staple triad. References to bread, wine, and olive oil can be found throughout classical writing, from the *Iliad* to the New Testament. To supplement these staples, Mediterranean people have traditionally eaten fish, fowl, goat cheese and yogurt (in those areas once part of the Turkish Empire), green vegetables and legumes (such as beans and peas), seasonal fruit, and garlic and onions.

We should emphasize here that the triad diet has never simply been a bland mush of starchy fillers wetted down with "greasy" olive oil and made palatable by large doses of wine. Anyone who has learned to enjoy traditional Mediterranean food will attest to its tasty diversity. Green vegetables have long played an important role in the traditional food of the region. But the vegetables had to be drought-resistant and had to have a long shelf-life without refrigeration. Also, kitchen-garden vegetables had to grow quickly on small rock-terrace patches of marginal soil. Wild spring greens and thistles were the forerunners of the cultivated spinach, cabbage, and broccoli now found in almost every Mediterranean kitchen-garden plot.

Beyond the triad staples and green vegetables, the traditional diet provides a variety of flavorful and nutritious components. Once again, these elements of the diet were determined by climatic imperatives. Garlic and onions ripen fast in the moist spring and dry well in the summer heat, as do peppers, lentils, and broad beans.

Fresh and dried fish were available throughout the year. Every coastal city had its fishing fleet, and most Mediterranean villages within a day's journey of the sea maintained a small "scala" or protected anchorage for open fishing boats. In the spring, when the wheat was ripening, the men fished for tuna and mackerel. On calm winter days, they netted bream and squid.

But red meat—especially the fatty, grain-fed beef and pork of northern Europe and America—has been notably absent from traditional Mediterranean cuisine. The region has never produced adequate year-round pasturage or fodder for large cattle herds. In the Roman republic, the ability to feed cattle on grain stubble was considered a revolutionary innovation, but the Mediterranean region has traditionally never had surplus grain adequate to produce the "marbled" meats available in northern Europe and North America. Even swine have been difficult to raise in many Mediterranean countries, and pork spoils quickly in the hot climate and is the vector of trichinosis, which might partially account for the Jewish and

Islamic aversion to this meat. Sheep and goats are the traditional meat animals of the region; but because they provided wool and milk and were, therefore, worth more alive than as a source of food, they were slaughtered only on special occasions. The notable exception to this is the spring lamb and kid season. Male lambs and kids were, indeed, surplus and could be sold or eaten. It probably is no accident that both the Christian feast of Easter and the Muslim feast of Eid el-Kebir involve the ritual slaughter of lambs (or, in many cases, kids). Even today some "poor" Mediterranean farmers taste red meat and white bread only once a year during their Easter banquet.

This traditional diet is also low in milk and butter, refined flour and sugar, and distilled liquor (distilling hard spirits requires large quantities of fuel, a perennially scarce commodity in the deforested Mediterranean).

Before proceeding further, we shall define some terms used throughout the book. For convenience' sake, we've often referred to traditional Mediterranean food as a "village" diet because this nutritional pattern is best preserved today in those small towns and villages that have not enjoyed the dubious "benefits" of contemporary affluence. We do not mean to imply that village food is bland, unrefined, or spartan. And, strictly speaking, many standard Mediterranean dishes did not originate in villages at all, but rather in working-class sections of cities such as Naples, Marseilles, Athens, and Valencia.

Most Mediterranean cities have a common link to the Roman Empire. During the Pax Romana, urban populations swelled with working people. While patricians dined on exotic luxuries, the urban poor relied on the staples of the traditional triad. Like their village cousins, city workers were forced by poverty to follow a moderate diet. Over the centuries, this diet has been steadily refined to include classic dishes of true elegance. Much of this evolution was sparked by fierce competition among market-place and neighborhood restaurants—the forerunners of today's tavernas and trattorias—for the patronage of city working people.

Thus, the humble origins of such dishes as pizza, paella, and bouillabaisse have been buried over centuries of refinement. Linguine con vongole may have been created by a humble clam-monger, but it is served today in Italy's best restaurants. In paella, one makes use of small pieces of fish and chicken, but these "scraps" are carefully selected and combined. Traditional Mediterranean food is rich in seasonings and spices that are so delicately incorporated in the cooking that the flavorful essence of the fresh ingredients is preserved.

As this cuisine evolved, it was accepted by both urban upper classes and by villagers, who adapted the cooking of the market-place inns and food stalls to their own kitchens. But, despite its long evolution, traditional Mediterranean food still relies on the fresh, simple bounty of local land and sea. And, as we shall see, it is this that provides the diet's health benefits.

The traditional diet's daily meals might include a breakfast of fresh or dried fruit, whole-grain bread, and yogurt. Lunch and dinner also emphasize cereals in the form of whole-grain bread or pasta. Fresh vegetables such as cabbage, spinach, kale, and broccoli are eaten almost every day. And olive oil—not red meat or dairy products —provides most of the daily fat intake. Wine usually accompanies both the midday and evening meals, but in small quantities—a glass or two for each adult. Fish provide most of this diet's animal protein, and garlic and onions flavor many dishes.

To the affluent eye, the lack of meat and the small amount of dairy products, plus the abundance of whole-grain cereals, olive oil, and garlic—foods we often ignore—are alien. In fact, researchers have found that up to 80 percent of the daily calories in the traditional Mediterranean diet are provided in the form of cereals and olive oil. In the affluent world, almost two-thirds of our daily calories come from animal fats and meat protein.

To understand better the foods that traditional Mediterranean villagers eat, we would like to describe a meal we shared last year with some friends on the Greek island of Rhodes, where we have been fortunate enough to have had a home for the past sixteen years.

This family gathering took place in the fishing village of Haráki, but it could have been duplicated almost anywhere in the Mediterranean. The Kostaki family was celebrating the name day of their beloved Yaya Eleni, the eighty-year-old matriarch of this large village clan, and was kind enough to invite us to join the group. On a cloudless, breezy afternoon, over two-dozen relatives met at Pavlo's seaside taverna.

Under the cane sunshade of the terrace, the women arranged clay bowls and cloth-covered pans, which held the food that they had contributed to the family feast. Wicker-covered wine jugs stood at strategic locations on the tables. Once the throng had been seated, Pavlo served platters of grilled barbounia—red mullet that he had pulled from his nets at dawn. At Grandma Eleni's table, Pavlo placed a beautifully grilled synagrida (gray snapper) before her.

Amid cries of "Bravo," the women uncovered their own dishes. Occupying the center of each table were large "horiatiki" (village) salads—colorful mounds of sliced tomatoes and cucumbers, garnished with wedges of white onions and shredded cabbage. As the children watched hungrily, a woman dressed the salads with generous amounts of olive oil. Once red-wine vinegar had been added to the salad dressing, children and adults alike dug into the bowls, using hunks of crusty whole-grain bread—fresh from the village ovens— to soak up the salad dressing.

As each dish of stuffed grape leaves or baked eggplant emerged from its cloth wrapper, the laughter and animated talk grew louder. In Greece, as elsewhere in the Mediterranean Basin, a meal is a social occasion, a time to relax with family and enjoy the bounty of the soil. Soon the plates were stacked with dolmádes and yemista—stuffed tomatoes, peppers, and zucchini, the rice filling enriched with currants, mint, and cinnamon. Aunt Marietta made a circuit of the tables, bearing a copper kettle of yigantes—broad beans cooked with olive oil, garlic, and tomatoes. Her sister Tsampika passed around a pot of boiled spinach dressed with olive oil and lemon juice.

A cool breeze rustled the cane roof and raised whitecaps out to sea. Piles of fishbones grew beside the plates (Greeks literally "dig in" with their hands when it comes to fresh fish, picking each fish frame clean of succulent morsels). Wine glasses were refilled, and adults toasted Eleni's health and the family's prosperity. When the last salad bowl was wiped clean with the last crust of bread and the last stuffed grape leaf had been eaten, the men left the tables to bring back baskets of fresh peaches and apricots from the spring beside the chapel, where the fruit had been cooling. Uncle Yiannis cut up yellow melons and striped watermelons, and added them to the mounds of fruit.

Those children who hadn't already been put on pallets to rest swooped down on the apricots and peaches. The adults, chatting quietly now, lingered over their wine and thimble-sized cups of Greek coffee. Later, young Dimitri would play his bouzouki, and there would be dancing. Now a short sleep was in order.

We were feeling drowsy ourselves and were casting covetous glances at choice shady spots along the sea wall where we might stretch out for a snooze. But then we noticed some newcomers on the taverna terrace. At another table, a family of English tourists from nearby Lindos had arrived for a late Sunday lunch. Pavlo offered them a choice of fresh bream and the red mullet that he'd served to the Kostaki family. But the tourists were not interested in his traditional dishes. The teen-aged daughter and the younger boy were sunburned and tired from a long morning on the beach. Perhaps they felt awkward in the presence of the large group of "foreigners" at the nearby tables. Furthermore, the parallel rows of gleaming fish eyes staring up at them from Pavlo's refrigerator case did not provoke uncontrollable spasms of appetite in the two children, who had probably never seen a fish with its head attached. So the father —stocky, middle-class—suggested a "nice fry-up": fried eggs, Danish bacon, and those German sausages they noticed in Pavlo's refrigerator.

The prospect of familiar food seemed to cheer the two youngsters. Pavlo offered a Greek village salad, but they preferred their tomatoes fried "in with the bacon." They chose small white sandwich rolls, not the crusty, whole-grain village bread, to accompany their meal.

Pavlo watched with a bemused smile. Over the years, he has learned to cater to the tastes of northern tourists. Now, thanks to the cornucopia obtainable through the Common Market, he has a dependable supply of bacon, sausage, pork, and beef, as well as Danish butter and Dutch cheese. But, like many Mediterranean villagers, he prefers the traditional diet he was raised on. Pavlo doesn't have much formal education, but he once told us he feels that a diet so rich in fatty meat and so poor in vegetables cannot be healthy.

The August sun set behind the island's granite shoulder. On the tables of Pavlo's taverna, the Kostaki women prepared a light dinner of mézéthes, small plates of beans, olives, spinach pastries, and cold vegetable dishes dressed with olive oil and garlic. Pavlo brought out a platter of grilled sardines. At the head table, Eleni gripped a knife in her strong, gnarled hand to cut the loaf she had baked before the sun rose that morning.

Young Dimitri finished a song and lay aside his bouzouki to lift a glass of wine. "Stini yia' sou," he toasted his grandmother—"To your health."

CHAPTER 2

Diet and Health in the Mediterranean World

It would be nice to be able to report that people all across the Mediterranean world still eat like the Kostaki clan at the name-day celebration for Grandma Eleni. But the unfortunate truth is that millions of people in Greek, Italian, and Spanish cities have abandoned traditional village food in favor of a more "affluent," meat-rich, low-carbohydrate diet. Ironically, as we shall see, this shift in eating habits has provided dramatic evidence (in the form of increased heart disease and cancer) of the health benefits of the traditional diet.[1]

It bears repeating, however, that even when the traditional Mediterranean diet is skewed toward a more affluent pattern, there seem to be certain components that continue to offer their protective qualities: whole grains, olive oil, wine, dark green and yellow "cruciferous" vegetables, fish, and garlic and onions.

It is easy enough to make this claim. After all, we've lived in the Mediterranean world for twenty years and have certainly gone native as far as our own diet is concerned. But, as we discovered while doing our research, such a claim is difficult to prove, especially to the satisfaction of skeptical health-organization bureaucrats. Fortunately, the medical discipline of epidemiology, which deals with the incidence, distribution, and control of diseases in entire populations, has come of age. It is a science of comparative information and is flourishing in this "age of information" in which high-speed computers can process enormous amounts of data. Whereas even ten years ago it would have been difficult to compare the relative combined incidence and distribution of cardiovascular disease and gastrointestinal cancers among the different countries of the world, medical statisticians can now electronically swap and match whole batches of information and, in the process, compare rural and urban regions within a country to similar regions elsewhere. And in the course of this recent research, there have been some interesting discoveries.[2]

For example, white Americans are among the most affluent people in the world. America has the most technically advanced health-care system on earth, with universal vaccination against infant and childhood diseases, the world's best sanitation and public hygiene systems, and a rapidly increasing level of health awareness among an almost universally educated population. Therefore, one would expect the life expectancy of white American men—the "elite" of our society —to be much higher than, say, that of Italian and Greek men.

Not true. The life expectancy of Italian men is 73.0 years; of Greek men, 72.2 years; and of white American men, 71.8 years.[3] Yet Greek and Italian men smoke more heavily than their American counterparts, despite the devastation smoking brings in the form of increased heart disease and cancer. Also, as anyone who has lived in both Greece and Italy can attest, the level of health care in these countries—especially in the rural areas, where large segments of the population still live—cannot compare to that in the United States. Furthermore, Greece and Italy were ravaged by World War II, and the men currently living to an average age of 73 experienced widespread famine and epidemics of infectious disease in the 1940s. In Greece, the terrible years of the war continued until 1949, as the people fought their bitter civil war. Thus, Italian and Greek men who are now in their sixties and seventies almost universally suffered more malnutrition and risk of infectious disease than their American contemporaries. And the improvements in sanitation, hygiene, and public-health care in the rural areas of these countries have only come about in the past twenty years.

What are the Greeks and Italians doing to live so long, or what *aren't* they doing?

Before answering that question, here are more statistics.

Heart attacks (called acute myocardial infarctions by health statisticians) kill an estimated 550,000 Americans every year. All told, about 1 million Americans die annually from cardiovascular disease.[4] Epidemiologists compute the incidence of a disease in a large population by its age-adjusted per-100,000 death rate for that particular affliction. According to the World Health Organization's most recent *Statistical Annual,* the current American per-100,000 heart-attack death rate is 132; in Italy, it is 74; and in Greece, it is 76. You don't have to be a mathematical genius to realize that the incidence of fatal heart attacks in America is roughly twice that of Italy and Greece.

Now let's look at the figures for colon cancer, which kills about 60,000 Americans each year. Our per-100,000 death rate is currently 19.5; in Italy, it is 11.4; and in Greece, it is 8.0.

The breast-cancer death rate for American women stands at 27.0 per 100,000; for Italian women, it is 22.3 per 100,000; and for Greek women, it is only 16.2 per 100,000.[5]

Yet the Italian statistics can be deceptive since Italy is culturally two separate countries: the affluent industrial north and the Mediterranean south.

When we asked WHO epidemiologist Dr. James Hanley to help us compare the different rates of cardiovascular disease and gastrointestinal cancers between the north of Italy and the Mediterranean south (where the traditional diet still prevails), what we discovered was fascinating. The highest per-100,000 death rates for these diseases (both combined and separately) occurred in the north, where the people follow a diet rich in meat and animal fats and are much more affluent than in the south. The lowest death rates occurred in two of the most traditionally Mediterranean provinces: Puglia, on the heel of the Italian boot, and Sardinia. In fact, the highest incidence of gastrointestinal cancers (79 deaths per 100,000) and cardiovascular disease (640 per 100,000) occurred in the Ligurian region of the industrial north; these rates were roughly double those of Puglia (gastrointestinal cancers: 31 per 100,000; cardiovascular disease: 380 per 100,000). Furthermore, there was a consistent north-south decline in the disease rates, with the meat-and-butter-rich north having the highest rates and the fish-pasta-and-olive-oil south the lowest.[6]

Seen in this light, the health benefits of the traditional Mediterranean triad diet become compelling. And when we return to Greece, the European country with the greatest proportion of its population still following the traditional diet, we are further convinced of the diet's protective qualities.

Dr. Christos Aravanis is an elderly, urbane physician, fluent in four languages. The tall, silver-haired professor is known as the dean of Greek cardiologists. At his office on central Athens's fashionable Queen Sofias Avenue, he treats a diverse group of patients, ranging from the capital's political and business elite to taxi drivers and longshoremen from Piraeus. His resident students in the Department of Cardiology at the Evangelismos Hospital Medical Center consider themselves privileged to study under Aravanis because he reputedly knows more about heart disease than any other doctor in Greece.

Yet fifty years ago, when Aravanis was a young physician completing his studies in Athens, he *never* saw a heart-attack patient. It was only after he came to the United States for advanced cardiology training that he witnessed his first acute myocardial infarction. He then realized that there was something in the Greek pattern of life —possibly in the traditional diet—that seemed to protect people from cardiovascular disease, which was assuming epidemic proportions in America in the 1940s.

Since then, Aravanis has been in the forefront of research dealing with the relationship between diet and heart disease in Greece. Starting in 1960, he and his colleague Dr. Paul Ioannidis led a seminal twenty-year research project: "Nutritional Factors and Cardiovascular Diseases in the Greek Island Heart Study,"[7] a so-called "cohort study," in which two demographically similar groups in separate locations were studied during the same period. This research traced the cardiovascular health of two cohorts of Greek island village men.

Crete and Corfu were chosen for study because the two islands were accessible from Athens and had homogeneous populations who basically ate the traditional Mediterranean diet. The Cretan group, from 12 villages, included 686 men aged 40 to 59 in 1960. The cohort from Corfu consisted of 529 men of the same age group from villages on the north coast. At the beginning, middle, and end of the study, the doctors, working with a team of research assistants, collected hundreds of daily food samples from the homes of the villagers. They also took detailed medical histories of the subjects.[8]

Each year, a team of expert physicians from Athens visited the villages, rigorously scrutinized the death records, questioned local doctors, and discussed the deaths with family members. The researchers were thus able to establish the exact cause of death of each of the deceased. For the purposes of the study, cardiovascular disease was broken down into two subcategories: ischemic heart disease (coronary heart disease, heart attacks, etc.) and cerebrovascular accidents (stroke). All other deaths were divided between cancers and "other causes."

At the beginning of the study in 1960, the researchers noted several small but possibly significant differences between the average daily diets of the Cretans and Corfiots. The average total daily caloric intake in the Corfu villages was around 3,000, while the village men of Crete averaged about 2,700 calories. Following the traditional Mediterranean pattern, both groups got most of their daily calories in the form of carbohydrates (bread or pasta) and vegetable fats (primarily olive oil). But the men on Corfu ate more protein (in the form of meat), consumed less olive oil, and drank more alcohol.

The differences in diet were not surprising. Corfu had been colonized by both the Italians and the British. A more affluent, less typically Mediterranean life style prevailed, even in the isolated villages of the north coast. Crete, however, was quintessentially Mediterranean. In 1960, the Cretan villagers survived basically on subsistence agriculture and remittance money from relatives who had emigrated. The Cretans received almost 90 percent of their daily calories in the form of carbohydrates and olive oil; their daily alcohol consumption amounted to one or two glasses of wine. In fact, these villagers were living examples of the Mediterranean's age-old dependence on the triad of wheat, olive, and grapes. Another important difference was that the Cretan villagers consumed home-baked whole-grain bread, while the Corfiots had begun to rely on commercially baked white bread.

During the twenty years of the study, Corfu's affluence steadily increased with the postwar tourist boom. Crete's economy also prospered, but more slowly. The packaged-tour invasion reached Crete later, and the relative affluence brought by the tourists' Deutsche marks and dollars was a long time coming to the Cretan villages in the study.

By the time the study was completed in 1980, both groups had increased their total average daily caloric intake. The men of Corfu had reached a daily average of almost 3,600 calories, the Cretans just over 3,000. And the Corfiots were following Helsing's predicted pattern: they had dramatically increased their consumption of meat, saturated fat, and alcohol, while the proportion of olive oil in their daily diet dropped from 25 percent to 16 percent. The Cretans also increased their meat and saturated-fat consumption, but proportionally less than did their counterparts on Corfu. And on Crete, the men had also reduced their olive-oil consumption: from 32 percent of daily calories in 1960 to only 18 percent in 1980. Although the caloric-percentage difference between the two groups' olive-oil consumption was insignificant at the end of the study, the Cretans consumed approximately one-third more olive oil than the Corfiots for a significant period.

On the whole, however, the relative poverty of the Cretans, vis-à-vis their counterparts on Corfu, forced them to maintain the moderation of the Mediterranean diet.

When the researchers totaled the twenty-year mortality rates for the two groups, they discovered significant differences. Using the statisical yardstick of death rates per 1,000 population (the standard small-population measurement), they found that the ischemic heart-disease death rate on Crete increased from 1.46 per 1,000 in 1961 to 13 per 1,000 in 1980. On Corfu, the heart-disease death rate almost tripled, from 13 per 1,000 in 1961 to just over 34 per 1,000 in 1980.

Comparing the death rate for stroke (cerebrovascular accident or CVA) in the two groups, the researchers discovered that between 1961 and 1980 the Cretan rate jumped from 1.46 to 32 per 1,000, while on Corfu the rate quadrupled, from 13 to 52 per 1,000.

Total cardiovascular-disease death rate by the end of the study was 45 per 1,000 on Crete and 86 per 1,000 on Corfu.

In other words, the affluent villagers on Corfu were dying from cardiovascular disease at almost *double* the rate of the more traditional men in the Cretan villages.

Cancer death rates for the two groups proportionally remained about the same, slowly rising on both islands as overall affluence increased. By 1980, the cancer death rate had actually decreased slightly on Corfu, probably due to improved local medical care.

As both groups became more affluent, the amount of rigorous daily activity declined. But each cohort still worked the fields and olive groves in the traditional manner, which involved walking several miles a day over steep country. At the end of their analysis, which used internationally accepted statistical methods, Aravanis's team concluded that the main difference between the two cohorts was diet. Although it is obvious that the entire group aged during the twenty-year study, the researchers assessed nutritional data for significant intracohort differences on an annual basis. Therefore, total-group aging was factored into the final analysis. (Those interested in the statistical methods employed in this study should consult the Notes at the end of this book.)[9]

The specific dietary factors that account for the striking difference in cardiovascular death rates between the two groups are interesting.

The *proportion* of olive oil to total daily calories seemed to offer the Cretans protection from cardiovascular disease. For the Corfiots, the increase of saturated fats in the form of dairy products and red meat, and the relative decrease in olive oil and carbohydrates, appeared to account for their decline in cardiovascular health. In other words, the village men on Corfu became victims of the deadly "disease of affluence" when they modified the traditional diet of their Mediterranean culture and partially embraced what British writer Anthony Burgess has so aptly dubbed the "cream and suet" diet of the northern Europeans.

What is interesting about this study is that, by the end of the research period in 1980, the diets of the villagers from Corfu and from Crete were not radically different from one another. But their diets differed in certain key aspects. Although the Cretans were eating more meat and saturated fats in 1980 than they did in 1961, their total daily calories were lower than the daily calorie intake of the Corfiots, and the Cretan villagers had not adopted the beer-and-hard-liquor drinking habits of the affluent Corfu villagers. As the food-calorie breakdown of the study shows, the Cretan villagers had maintained the moderate wine-with-meals pattern of the traditional Mediterranean diet. In addition to the proportion of olive oil in the Cretan diet, this moderate wine consumption might well have protected the Cretan men as much as certain other components of their diet.[10]

The men on Corfu had only added about 600 calories to their daily total average, but they suffered a cardiovascular-disease death rate almost twice as high as their counterparts on Crete. Therefore, the role of olive oil in the traditional Mediterranean diet, which was another key difference that the researchers found between the two groups, becomes increasingly important and is a subject we will explore later.

Another recent Greek study concerns the role of the Mediterranean diet in protecting people from colorectal cancer, the Number 2 cause of cancer death in the United States. In 1980, a team of Greek and British physicians carried out a so-called "case control" study in which 100 consecutive colorectal cancer patients at two Athens hospitals—the "cases"—were matched by age and sex with 100 cancer-free orthopedic patients—the "controls"—in the same hospitals.[11] Once the patients' complete medical histories were taken, the researchers conducted detailed surveys of the patients' dietary habits. Eighty food items in nine main categories were listed, and the cancer patients and their matched controls were asked to list carefully the number of times per week they normally ate these items.

The study's nine food groups were:

- *Cereals*—including white and whole-grain breads, pasta, rice, etc.
- *Starchy roots*—potatoes
- *Refined sugars*—jellies, baked sweets, glacéed fruit, etc.
- *Pulses, nuts, and seeds*—green beans, broad beans, chickpeas, lentils, etc.
- *Vegetables*—tomatoes, cucumbers, cabbage, spinach, broccoli, cauliflower, etc.
- *Fruits*—melons, apricots, apples, peaches, etc.
- *Meat, fish, and eggs*—pork, beef, veal, lamb, goat, fish, and eggs
- *Dairy products*—cheese, whole milk, yogurt, ice cream
- *Oils and fats*—butter, whole olives, olive oil

The researchers immediately noticed a "substantial nutritional variability" in the population of Athens. In other words, many people were following the traditional Mediterranean diet, while others had adopted an almost totally affluent pattern of eating. This created a "favorable situation for a case-control epidemiological investigation of the nutritional causes of disease."

When the diet statistics were tabulated and subjected to rigorous standard analyses, the researchers found clear evidence that the traditional Mediterranean diet protected the control group, whereas the more "Western" the diet of the patients became, the greater the incidence of colorectal cancer.[12]

Those with cancer reported significantly less frequent consumption of vegetables, especially cruciferous vegetables—beets, spinach, and cabbage—which traditionally supplement the basic triad diet. As an independent factor, the cancer victims also reported significantly more frequent consumption of meat, especially of beef and lamb. The control group reported relatively low-meat and high-vegetable consumption, with some controls following the almost meatless high-carbohydrate and high–olive-oil diet traditional to the area.

Between the two extremes of the high-meat, low-vegetable, low-fiber "Western" dietary pattern of those with cancer and the low-meat, high-vegetable, and high-fiber "Mediterranean" pattern of the controls, there was a startling eightfold risk ratio. In other words, those with cancer who had abandoned their traditional diet for the affluent Western diet were eight times as likely as the control group to develop colorectal cancer.[13] Equally important, those who followed the traditional diet, especially in regard to daily fruit and vegetable consumption, and who almost totally abstained from eating red meat seemed to enjoy an eightfold protective factor from this disease. These results are consistent with the Italian north-south gastrointestinal cancer-incidence pattern we observed earlier.[14]

Follow-up studies in Greece and elsewhere in the Mediterranean support the major findings of the 1980 case-control cancer study.[15] This research has led one of Greece's leading nutritional experts, Dr. Antonia Trichopoulou, to study the relationship between her country's growing affluence—and its changing pattern of diet—and the changes in disease incidence.[16]

Trichopoulou carefully surveyed Greek dietary patterns between

1960 and 1980, the same period covered by the Crete-Corfu cardio-vascular-disease study. She then tabulated the changing pattern of disease incidence for these two decades.

The food groups she studied were basically the same as the categories in the cancer case-control research project: meat, fish, eggs, dairy products, cereals, beans, vegetables, fruits, and sugar. Her findings were predictable, based on Helsing's model of affluent malnutrition, but still offer dramatic proof of the rapid dietary changes currently affecting the traditional Mediterranean world.

Between 1960 and 1975, for example, Greeks ate an annual per-capita average of less then 30 kilograms of meat, which placed them far below the Americans and northern Europeans for the same period; by 1980, however, Greeks were averaging 70 kilograms of meat each year—an increase of 133 percent over 1960—and they were approaching the average annual per-capita meat consumption of their Common Market neighbors. Greek consumption of dairy products jumped 82 percent between 1960 and 1980. Egg consumption shot up 50 percent in the same period. For sugar, the figures are equally dramatic: a 106-percent increase during the two decades.

Those food items that the Greeks consumed in lesser quantities over the two-decade period are equally illuminating: fish—down 4 percent; cereal grains—down 15 percent; beans, peas, etc.—down 28 percent. And consumption of fruit and vegetables increased only marginally during the twenty years studied.

Overall daily average calories consumed rose by 16 percent, and this was mostly in the form of meat and saturated animal fats. In fact, total animal-fat consumption had increased 71 percent by 1980.[17]

When she turned to the changing pattern of disease incidence in Greece for the same two decades, Trichopoulou found convincing evidence of the diet-disease link. In 1969, coronary-heart-disease (CHD) incidence was so low in Greece that a number of international researchers investigated the Greek diet and life style.[18] But by 1980, the CHD death rate had shot up dramatically. Although still far below the CHD death rates for industrial northern Europe and the United States, the Greek CHD death rate for men climbed above that of France in 1975 and is still rising.[19] This steady increase in CHD among Greek adults coincides with an equally steady increase in serum cholesterol, especially among affluent city dwellers.[20]

When Trichopoulou turned to the health indices of Greek children, she found an "ominous" trend: both hypertension and obesity, precursors of CHD, were rapidly increasing among affluent urban children.[21]

The pattern was similar for the age-adjusted death rates due to colorectal and breast cancers. "In both these cancers," Trichopoulou states, "the time trends are increasing in a steady and almost alarming way."

Next, Trichopoulou compared the death rates for diabetes mellitus for both urban and rural areas. Diabetes onset, Trichopoulou states, may be closely connected to diet.[22] Although other factors such as pregnancy, genetic predisposition, and pancreatic impairment due to viral diseases are also causes of diabetes onset, grossly immoderate diet, which overloads the metabolic function of the pancreas, is widely assumed to be a major cause of diabetes.[23] Therefore, the disease death rates could indicate the impact of the increasingly popular "Western" diet in Greece.

Not surprisingly, in the course of her research, Trichopoulou discovered that the diabetes death rate for villagers who followed the traditional diet was less than one-third that of city dwellers who had forgone this diet.

Presented with such evidence of the connection between diet and disease, and of the protective value of the traditionally moderate Mediterranean diet, leading physicians like Aravanis and Trichopoulou have pioneered nutritional education campaigns in Greece. When Aravanis addresses medical students today in Athens, he gives them an unequivocal message: "You *must* tell your patients to return to the diet of their great-grandfathers in the villages." He and Trichopoulou have worked with other medical leaders to convince government officials of the dangers of the affluent Western diet. Like in many European countries, the Greek government controls the prices and production levels of certain basic food commodities: flour, fish, dairy products, etc. After Greece joined the Common Market, that country was pressured by fellow members to purchase an enormous amount of cheap meat and dairy products. At the same time, there was increased domestic demand for white bread and baked goods made with refined flour. In short, the combination of Common Market surpluses and changing domestic tastes were steadily driving Greek city dwellers away from their traditional diet.

But the leaders of the medical community lobbied hard for price controls and increased production of whole-grain bread in the country's subsidized bakeries. Then they turned to the question of cheap butter and animal shortening, which were rapidly replacing olive oil. To help better educate the public, the doctors convinced the government to carry out a televised campaign on the benefits of olive oil compared to saturated animal fats. This shift from inexpensive government-subsidized butter and back to olive oil may save tens of thousands of lives in the years to come.

But before we examine the specific advantages of olive oil, whole grain, wine, and the other key components of the traditional Mediterranean diet, we should briefly consider what medical research has recently established about the actual mechanics of the connection between diet and disease.

C H A P T E R   3

Diet and Disease:
What Science Knows

In most parts of the world, the scientific establishment resides within a hierarchical research bureaucracy. And, as people from Shanghai to Milwaukee can attest, bureaucracies are inherently conservative; they crawl—they do not leap—to conclusions. In this regard, medical research reflects the habits and attitudes of the larger scientific establishment. However, since medical and nutritional researchers are dealing with human lives, caution is often warranted.

Thus, endorsement of scientific evidence linking diet with cardiovascular disease and cancer has come very slowly from the world's collective medical-research establishment. But it has come.

In 1961, the American Heart Association issued guidelines *suggesting* "the possible relation of dietary fat to heart attacks and stroke."[1] Many Americans learned for the first time that there was a connection between the levels of a substance in our blood called serum cholesterol and increased risk of heart disease. That was twenty-five years ago. Each year since then, about 1 million Americans have died of cardiovascular disease. Awareness of the problem has dawned slowly on the mass of otherwise well-educated Americans. And epidemic heart disease has not dropped as quickly as it should have. In some communities of America's industrial Northeast, for example, 1 in 4 males over age 55 has heart disease.[2]

And some sectors of the medical research establishment are still debating the link between blood cholesterol and heart disease. But the majority of medical experts, including the Expert Committee on Cardiovascular Disease of the World Health Organization, now insist that there is a direct link between blood cholesterol and heart disease.[3]

Meanwhile, the great mass of us muddle along, worrying about pollution, the bomb, our waistlines, and the mortgage. Almost everyone we know (ourselves included) spends a few moments a day thinking about ways to stay healthy. Most of us are terrified of cancer, yet how many of us realize that fewer than half as many Americans die each year of cancer than of heart disease? Nevertheless, cancer is the Number 2 killer disease in America, so there is good reason to be worried. But were we ever taught in school that there is scientific evidence linking certain common cancers and diet? We now know that dietary fiber is good for us, but that news was a long time coming from the medical establishment.

Although this is not a scientific study, we do know how to read in several languages and can tot up a column of statistics with the best of them. We want you to consider what medical research has discovered to date about the diet-disease connection, to form your own conclusions, and to keep those conclusions in mind as you read the rest of this book.

First, we should define two key terms.

Triglycerides. This term confuses many people because doctors often talk of serum triglyceride levels in ominous tones. Basically, *triglyceride* describes dietary fat; it is a compound in which three fatty-acid molecules are linked. In this book, we are more interested in specific types of fatty acid—the serum lipids—and, even more specifically, the metabolic products of these lipids—namely, cholesterol. Therefore, we will not use the term *triglycerides* often.

Cholesterol. Everybody has heard of it; most of us think it is "bad"; yet few of us could write a simple definition of the word, and fewer still could describe in plain language the function of this substance within the human body.

Recently, we were in the Georgetown Safeway on a busy Saturday morning. It is the place for trendy, upscale young couples to shop, and the food on display reflects the tastes of the best-educated, best-paid people in the country, maybe in the world. In the aisle offering cooking oil, we encountered an attractive young couple in fashionably rumpled tennis togs. They were pondering the shelves of corn and safflower oils, seemingly involved in an important nutritional decision. Finally the young woman reached up with her lean, tanned arm and removed a hefty plastic jug of a popular corn oil.

"Look," she said with a knowing nod to her mate, then tapped the jug's label. "No Cholesterol," the label proclaimed in bold red type.

"All *right,*" the young man beamed, seizing the plastic bottle as if he'd just been handed a breakthrough in modern science.

As they pushed their cart down the aisle, it was clear that they felt good about their discovery of cholesterol-free cooking oil. Twenty years ago, only 1 person in 100 had heard of cholesterol; now it's a common household (not to mention Madison Avenue) word. But it was obvious that these well-educated people did not understand much about the substance.

Cholesterol is produced by *animal* tissue. It is an important constituent of animal cells. No vegetable oil on earth—corn, safflower, soybean, or olive—has ever contained a single milligram of cholesterol.

But this couple knew that cholesterol was "bad" for their health and were happy with their cleverly packaged corn oil. Their choice was emblematic of the linkage between increased health awareness and fundamental confusion about nutrition in general. We shake our heads sadly at the benighted Third World mothers who succumbed to the blandishments of Nestlé and abandoned breast feeding for infant formula, yet we ourselves eagerly buy cholesterol-free corn oil. But how would we react if there were a boldly printed sign above the Safeway's produce bins proclaiming "blood-free" apples and cucumbers?

Our ignorance of such biological fundamentals has not only nurtured confusion about nutrition and disease, but has prepared the way for the legions of quack diet books on the midway of the shopping-mall bookstores.

Getting back to cholesterol, it exists in all animal cells, including our own. When we eat animal food products, we ingest cholesterol. Certain animal foods have more cholesterol than others. An egg yolk, for example, has ten times as much cholesterol as an 8-ounce glass of whole milk. Besides eggs, the highest concentration of food cholesterol may be found in meat, liver, and some shellfish. The cholesterol content of animal foods, therefore—or *dietary cholesterol,* as medical researchers call it—is something with which we should be familiar.

But there is another kind of cholesterol—that which exists in our own bodies. This is known as *serum cholesterol* or *blood cholesterol.* We need it for normal growth and metabolism, and there is a tiny bit in every cell in our bodies. Cholesterol is produced in our liver as part of the digestive process. When we eat food high in cholesterol, however, such as eggs, whole milk, or red meat, our level of natural serum cholesterol increases beyond our normal metabolic needs.

To further complicate our examination, we must point out that pure chemical cholesterol is not simply "dissolved" in our blood to circulate like sugar in Kool Aid. The cholesterol that our bodies manufacture and that we eat is carried in our bloodstream by complex aggregate molecules called *lipoproteins,* combinations of fatty acids (lipids) and protein. And we have at least two kinds of these: *low-density lipoproteins* (LDLs) and *high-density lipoproteins* (HDLs).

LDLs carry most of the excess cholesterol our bodies cannot metabolize or eliminate and deposit this cholesterol on the walls of our bloodstream in the form of a fatty microscopic plaque. HDLs, on the other hand, tend to carry vital cholesterol to our tissues.

Therefore, LDLs have become known as "bad" cholesterol, and HDLs have acquired the title "good" cholesterol. Although certain medical scientists might find this definition simplistic, it provides the layperson with a useful tool for assessing nutrition.

Another term we should understand is *fat.* Fatty acids are found in both animal and vegetable foods: beef lard, bacon fat, fish oil, milk, corn oil, coconuts, and olive oil. The major difference among these fats is their degree of hydrogenation or their level of "saturation." A saturated fat's complex hydrocarbon molecular structure contains completely filled, or *saturated,* carbon-hydrogen bonds. Accordingly, it is difficult for such molecules to interact chemically during digestion and metabolism. In lay language, saturated fat is not easily broken down and "burned" during normal metabolism. We speak of fat being "stored" by the body, and, on the biochemical level, this is not a bad analogy.[4]

Most saturated fat is animal in origin. The degree of saturation can be easily noted by the physical properties of the fat in question. Saturated fats—butter, lard, bacon fat, etc.—remain solid at room temperature.

We've all heard of *polyunsaturated* fats—"cholesterol-free" corn oil is a prime example. These fats' hydrocarbon chains have many— or *poly-* —hydrogen openings. Therefore, they can interact chemically more readily during digestion and metabolism.

Finally, and most important for our study, we turn to *monounsaturated* fat. As the prefix *mono-* implies, there are only *one* or two places on the molecular structure of this kind of fat where hydrogen can bond. The most common monounsaturated fats are olive oil and peanut oil. However, there is a class of animal fats that have important polyunsaturates—the fish oils that contain omega-3 fatty acids —which we will discuss later in detail.

However, we must point out that all fats, from bacon grease to olive oil, are mixtures of saturated, polyunsaturated, and monounsaturated fatty-acid molecules, or lipids. We classify the fats according to their degree of hydrogen saturation.

What, then, is the relationship between the fats we eat and our level of serum cholesterol and lipoproteins? Saturated animal fats, especially the lard or tallowlike fats of "well-marbled" red meats, contain large amounts of cholesterol. When we eat such foods, the digestive process liberates high concentrations of cholesterol, and our body is stimulated to produce LDL carriers to transport this cholesterol throughout our system. Unfortunately, most of this cholesterol is deposited along the linings of our blood vessels. The resulting deposits harden and eventually block the blood vessel, a condition known as atherosclerosis. When a coronary artery is the affected blood vessel, a heart attack, or acute myocardial infarction, can result.[5]

In 1985, over 500,000 Americans died of this affliction, a casualty figure roughly equal to our battle deaths in World War II.[6] This carnage is so terrible that the perennially cautious medical research establishment has been shocked into action. In recent dietary guidelines, the American Heart Association made this unusually direct statement: "[Recent medical research has brought us] two well-established facts: dietary saturated fats and cholesterol directly raise the plasma total- and LDL-cholesterol, and high total- and LDL-cholesterol contribute directly to atherosclerosis and coronary heart disease."[7]

But such warnings haven't alarmed many Americans out of their bad dietary habits. Currently, Americans get about 40 percent of their daily calories as fats, of which almost half are saturated.[8] The main sources of these fats are meat, animal shortening, and dairy products.

This leads us to the other important element of this discussion: the relationship between diet and cancer. According to Dr. Oliver Alabaster, director of Cancer Research at George Washington University, "At least 35 percent of all cancer in the United States could be eliminated by simple changes in the nation's diet." He adds that as much as 60 percent of cancer in women and 40 percent of cancer in men have a dietary root-cause.[9] And the cause he pinpoints should not surprise us: high consumption of fats, especially the saturated animal fats found in meats. As we describe what science has discovered in recent years about the diet-cancer relationship, we should bear in mind the Athens colorectal cancer case-control study done in 1980. Almost all those Greeks who fell victim to this disease had abandoned their traditional village diet for "a Western pattern of nutrition."

In terms of the mechanics of the fat-cancer connection, it has been established that there *is* a link among levels of dietary fats, serum cholesterol, and certain cancers. Comparative epidemiological studies have consistently shown that a high-fat diet increases the incidence of breast, uterine, and ovarian cancer in women, prostate cancer in men, and cancer of the colon, liver, and pancreas in both sexes.[10] This is not a theoretical assumption, but a statistical absolute that holds true from Japan to America and Europe. And one should bear in mind that these cancers are among the deadliest forms of malignancies. The lung cancer that is provoked by tobacco use is deadlier; we are, however, learning the truth about tobacco. But breast and colorectal cancer are on the rise in the industrialized world, as lung cancer slowly drops with decreased smoking. And research that has tracked the increased incidence of breast and colorectal cancer has also cited a parallel dietary increase in meat and fat consumption.

The two most commonly accepted theories of dietary fat's carcinogenic role are both complex and controversial in that there is not yet a large body of human-subject research available to chart completely the biological mechanisms involved. One theory involves the role of fried, charbroiled, and roasted red meat. The high-temperature charring of fatty meats such as beef, lamb, and pork, the theory goes, produces carcinogenic compounds from the fats. These compounds, not easily digested, linger for long periods in the colorectal tract before elimination, thus provoking tumor formation in those tissues. To a certain degree, any fatty meat, no matter how it is prepared, presents this hazard because the waxy cholesterol that is found in animal fats can only be eliminated through the intestinal tract since it is not water-soluble and cannot pass through the urinary system. Therefore, the digestive products of cholesterol, known as bile acids, concentrate in the colon and rectum, where, by a chemical process not yet completely understood, they stimulate tumor formation.[11]

To make things more confusing, some recent studies have linked a diet high in polyunsaturates, like those found in many margarines, with certain cancers. This research is based on the assumption that the polyunsaturates liberate in the intestinal tract hydrocarbons known as *free radicals,* and that these molecules stimulate tumor formation. Many of these same researchers, however, state that the incidence of such cancer is much less than those provoked by the red-meat, bile-acid mechanism.[12]

Another theory deals with the role of a high-fat diet in stimulating hormones in the endocrine system, thus endangering those organs that are most sensitive to hormonal imbalances: breasts, ovaries, uterus, and prostate. Taking this theory one step further, researchers have found that the obesity often connected to a high-fat diet is a major factor in endocrine-induced cancers. According to Dr. Artemis Simopoulos, head of the nutrition coordinating committee of the National Institutes of Health, "Fat tissue is an endocrine system" that generates unnatural levels of hormones, including active estrogens. These high estrogen levels have been clearly linked to cancer of the cervix, breast, and uterus.[13]

And, as Trichopoulou also discovered in Greece, there is a link between increased dietary fat, obesity, and increased cancer risk.[14]

But, as Alabaster frankly admits, "if scientists knew how fats actually cause cancer, we would have a clearer understanding of the whole process of cancer formation." For the moment, however, he adds, science has not pinned down the exact mechanism. But this does not stop him from unequivocally warning us about dietary fat and cancer. In 1977, when the U.S. government called on Americans to reduce their level of dietary fat from 40 percent to 30 percent, Alabaster went a step further. Such recommendations are the product of cautious bureaucracies, he stressed. He urges Americans to reduce their fat intake to an average of only 20 percent of daily calories.[15]

In summary, the high levels of dietary fat in the industrialized Western world have been clearly linked to heart disease and cancer. A cursory survey of health statistics shows that in America these diseases have increased steadily with affluence during this century. While we are now seeing a leveling-off and drop of certain cardiovascular diseases in this country, the statistics for cancer are less encouraging. In fact, the *New England Journal of Medicine* recently published a paper that called the progress made to date in cancer treatment a "failure" and urged increased emphasis to be placed on cancer prevention, especially by educating the public about diet.[16]

Such public-education campaigns will not be easy. As we've seen, some parts of America have rates of cardiovascular disease that can only be described as epidemic among older citizens, especially among the traditional meat-and-potatoes men, aged 40 to 60. And the picture is not much brighter for many young people.[17] Researchers have found a startling level of cholesterol-induced atherosclerosis while performing autopsies on teen-aged accident victims, findings that coincide with autopsies performed on young servicemen killed in the Vietnam war. Most researchers attribute this discouraging news to the high-fat burger-and-shake diet favored by so many young people today. If Americans are ever going to lower their daily caloric fat intake to 20 percent, they are going to have to take a hard look at the fast-food industry.

Fast food is also partially responsible for the general overall increase in total daily calories consumed by Americans since World War II. When you examine the calories in a typical fast-food breakfast or lunch, including the large percentage of "empty" refined-carbohydrate calories, it is easy to see why. But every responsible public-health organization in the country urges Americans to reduce daily calories, thus reducing the proportions of the obesity epidemic plaguing us. To do so, we will have to take a hard look at our fast-food addiction.

Barely thirty years old, America's fast-food franchises now do $50-billion worth of business each year. And almost all this business is based on fatty foods: beef, fried chicken, and sweets. Only recently did McDonald's admit that they've been frying their fish fillets and chicken nuggets—their healthiest offerings—in beef tallow for years. Customers, they stated, like the taste. In other words, customers are addicted to high concentrations of animal fats. But, perhaps bending to the pressure of health-conscious Americans, McDonald's and other restaurant chains are now using more vegetable fats in their cooking.

And many of these customers are youngsters. If you divide the fast-food chains' $50 billion by our 230 million citizens, subtract the elderly in nursing homes and toothless infants, you'll see that adolescents and young adults are spending a per-capita average of almost $350 a year on fast foods. This works out to about six fast-food fixes a week. And what are they getting for their money?

According to the Washington-based Center for Science in the Public Interest, the most popular fast-food meals also contain the highest levels of saturated fats. For example:

- a double-beef Whopper at Burger King yields 12 teaspoons of saturated fat
- Wendy's triple cheeseburger produces 15 teaspoonfuls of saturated fats
- the Chicken McNuggets at McDonald's contain more fat than does McDonald's plain hamburger[18]

Americans are going to have to re-examine their eating habits and find different models of nutrition. And we feel that the model offered by the traditional Mediterranean diet presents the closest example we've yet seen of optimal nutrition.

PART II

The Food of the Mediterranean World

CHAPTER 4

Whole Grains and Cereals: The True Staff of Life

One of the most important components of the traditional Mediterranean diet is also the first part of the classical triad: grain. In this regard, the Mediterranean diet is similar to peasant diets found around the world. The Crete-Corfu study showed us that the villagers of southern Crete obtained more than 50 percent of their daily calories as complex carbohydrates, mainly in the form of stone-milled whole-wheat bread, baked daily at home in small fournos that stand like whitewashed beehives beside each house.

Other studies show that the southern Italians who had dramatically lower rates of cardiovascular disease and gastrointestinal cancer than their northern neighbors also had a much lower level of serum LDL cholesterol. These southern villagers received an average of 55 to 60 percent of their daily calories as complex carbohydrates—primarily bread and pasta—while the northern Italians received an average of less than 45 percent of daily calories in the form of mixed simple and complex carbohydrates.[1]

Before we proceed, we should define *simple carbohydrates* and *complex carbohydrates,* describing their role in human nutrition not only in the Mediterranean, but throughout the world.

Like fats, carbohydrates are organic molecules composed of life's principal chemical constituents: a core "chain" of carbon with atoms of hydrogen attached to one side of the chain and submolecules of oxygen-hydrogen (hydroxyls) attached to the other. Carbohydrates are a product of photosynthesis in plants, during which the hydrogen of the water in the plant is combined with atmospheric carbon dioxide. During this process, plants also liberate oxygen into the air. So we're not talking about some arcane biochemical curiosity, but rather about the fundamental continuum of life in our planet's biosphere.

The structure of carbohydrates is asymmetrical, which explains the bewildering variety of carbohydrates that have the same three elements in the same amounts but are geometrically dissimilar on the molecular level. Even given this variety, we may categorize carbohydrates in three groups: sugars, starch, and cellulose.

The simplest carbohydrates are the sugars such as glucose, a principal component of refined table sugar.

Starches are generally more complex. Most starch in the human diet comes from tubers and cereal grains, with the latter providing by far the bulk of human nutritional needs around the world. Indeed, complex grain carbohydrates provide more than 50 percent of the daily caloric intake for more than 50 percent of the people in the world. In Latin America, corn fills this role; in the Far East, rice is the staple; and from the Indian subcontinent through the Mediterranean Basin, the staple grain is wheat and the staple food has traditionally been stone-ground whole-wheat bread.

The nutritional advantages of complex carbohydrates from whole grains are threefold:

- The millstone crushes the wheat but does not remove the cellulose skin of the grain—that is, the bran, of which we have recently heard so much.
- The sprouting end of the grain kernel, called the germ, is a rich source of vitamins and protein.
- And the starchy center of the grain provides the complex carbohydrates that our body can efficiently convert into energy and the replacement compounds that support our complex cellular life.

Most of us in the West, however, would not consider as "balanced" a daily diet that provides 50 percent of its calories from starch. But before we allow our recently acquired meat-protein chauvinism to color our thinking about the "starchy" diets of Third World people, let's recall that most human beings have survived on diets low in meat and high in whole-grain carbohydrates since Neolithic times, 12,000 years ago. Their descendants are those healthy people who the WHO Expert Committee on Cardiovascular Disease said "are well nourished . . . and have a good life expectancy at all ages."[2]

It is *our* current diet that is unbalanced, not those of Chinese farmers, Indian peasants, and villagers in Calabria. Unfortunately, most Americans and Europeans do not have historical perspective from which to judge their current eating habits. We have become so affluent that we tend to eat on a daily basis food that was once considered banquet fare. And this immoderate approach to nutrition has fostered the diseases of affluence.

Unless we have traveled widely, most of us never get the chance to see how the rest of the world meets its nutritional needs. The meals we are served in a good Greek or Italian restaurant are made up of banquet food, rich in meat delicacies that villagers might eat once or twice a year. The same holds true for many of the dishes cooked in Chinese restaurants. Ironically, even the soul food that many American blacks consider a legitimate aspect of their Afro-American heritage is actually banquet food. Black slaves survived day in, day out on corn meal and greens; the pork dishes around which so much soul food is centered were only available on special occasions.

And how many of us recall that old nursery rhyme "Pease porridge hot, / Pease porridge cold, / Pease porridge in the pot, / Nine days old"? The daily porridge of the British peasant was a mixture of grain and legumes (peas). We don't find many nursery rhymes about char-broiled steaks or milk shakes, do we? And even in the United States, daily consumption of meat is a relatively recent phenomenon for the mass of our citizens. Bread, oatmeal, corn meal, dumplings, and noodles were far more prevalent in our national diet than they are today.

But our subject of interest is the role of whole grains and cereals in the Mediterranean diet. Traditional Mediterranean bread—the "daily bread" of the Bible—is made from stone-milled whole grain, usually wheat or barley. Ranging from the dark pita of the Levant through the crusty brown loaves of Sicily to the heavy khobz of Morocco, whole-grain bread accompanies almost every meal. And when cracked-grain dishes such as bulgur are considered, it becomes obvious that cereal foods form a major component of the diet.

Once dismissed by affluent Westerners as starchy fillers, complex carbohydrates are now recognized as an important source of B vitamins, iron, and vital dietary fiber (among other things) as well as compounds such as phytic acid, which shows evidence of inhibiting the formation of intestinal cancers. Researchers at Pillsbury and at the University of Minnesota have shown that the carcinogens that attack our intestinal tract as a result of a high-fat, high-meat diet depend on a chemical process called iron-catalyst lipid peroxidation. The high amount of phytic acid found in cereal foods inhibits this process, allowing the bran of the cereal to carry the carcinogens safely away before tumor formation can begin.[3]

Whereas in the traditional Mediterranean diet whole-grain foods and other cereals make up more than half the daily intake of calories, Americans currently take in only one-quarter of their daily calories as cereal grains, much of it in the form of refined-flour products having no bran or germ protein.[4] The balance of our carbohydrate consumption is in the form of vegetable starch and simple sugars. Combined with our current high levels of saturated fats, our collective sweet tooth might account for the alarming degree of obesity in the industrialized world today.

Contrary to popular belief, complex carbohydrates such as whole-grain cereal foods and pasta are not "fattening"; fats and sugars, not complex carbohydrates, add the inches to our waists and hips. Because they are slowly and completely digested, complex carbohydrates are more efficiently "burned" in the metabolic process than are fats and sugars. Simple carbohydrates (sugars), often called "empty calories," do not contribute to our daily nutrient needs, but simply increase obesity.[5] Ronald Reagan's jelly beans notwithstanding, candy is junk food. Yet the overweight citizens of the industrialized world eat billions of dollars worth of sugary sweets annually. Indeed, according to Jane Brody, nationally recognized nutritional expert, Americans currently consume almost 20 percent of their daily calories in the form of sugar.[6]

Alarmed by the steady rise in obesity in America, leading government nutritionists now urge Americans to replace the large proportion of fats and sugars in their diet with complex carbohydrates—that is, return to the diets of our own forefathers, just as Aravanis recommended to contemporary Greeks. Nutritionists suggest that we increase cereal-grain consumption because these foods contain important nutrients, have a low calorie density per unit volume, and offer an important psychological benefit—"satiety," or meal satisfaction. Cereal grains, they say, can protect us from overconsumption of high-calorie (but low-density) fatty meats and rich desserts.[7]

But the American Heart Association has an even more compelling reason for urging Americans to eat more complex carbohydrates. When we replace the saturated fats of meats with carbohydrates, our level of "bad" LDL cholesterol drops, but not the HDL needed for good health. Joining other nutritional experts, the AHA suggests that Americans follow the pattern of southern Italian and Greek villagers, and increase complex-carbohydrate consumption to 55 percent of total daily calories.[8]

If this increase takes the form of whole-grain foods, we will also benefit from an increased intake of vital dietary fiber and important vegetable protein. The cellulose fiber of bran "keeps our insides working well," to paraphrase a popular TV commercial. Research studies have repeatedly shown that daily voiding of the intestinal tract (that is, regularity) carries away the carcinogenic residue—the bile acids—resulting from saturated-fat and meat consumption.[9] It is important to bear in mind that fats are *not* water-soluble; the only way we can eliminate the excess metabolic fat products is through our intestines. Chronic constipation is, indeed, a "disaster," to quote yet another TV commercial. And, judging from the hundreds of millions of dollars Americans spend each year on laxatives, it's a disaster experienced by a large proportion of our population.

But, amid all the confusing claims of cereal manufacturers and popular nutrition gurus, bear in mind these simple facts: high-fat, high-meat, low-fiber diets have been directly linked to colorectal cancer, but daily consumption of whole-grain foods (as shown in the Athens case-control study) can offer protection.[10]

Pasta, although not a whole-grain cereal food (it is made from the hard durum wheat native to the Mediterranean Basin), is very attractive to the nutritionist. Durum wheat is loaded with high-quality complex carbohydrates and has a surprisingly high percentage of protein (almost 20 percent for some varieties). But, as noted above, pasta is a high-volume, low-calorie food. The usable nutrition and the satisfaction derived from eating a pasta meal such as linguine with olive oil and garlic come without consumption of excess calories, saturated fats, and cholesterol. In the traditional Mediterranean village diet, pasta will often replace whole-grain bread in one daily meal. For instance, pasta may be added to protein-rich beans and peas in minestrone-type soups.

Before we leave the subject of complex carbohydrates in the traditional Mediterranean diet, we should touch on peas and beans. Beans, peas, chickpeas, and lentils belong to a class of vegetables known as legumes. They are high in protein, contain no saturated fat, and provide healthy amounts of complex carbohydrates. References to legumes can be found throughout classical literature: the Biblical Esau, who traded his wealth for a bowl of "pottage," probably received a meal of lentils. And legumes are found in many varieties in traditional Mediterranean food.

Studies show that the water-soluble fiber in legumes slows LDL-cholesterol production in the liver and also helps remove excess serum-LDL. In addition, this fiber speeds elimination and, because it is water-soluble, can "scavenge" for LDL plaque more efficiently than the insoluble fiber of grain bran.[11]

Finally, the vegetable protein found in peas and beans combines well with the protein and starch of complex carbohydrates to provide the right amino acids we need for good metabolism and growth. In some parts of the Mediterranean world, especially in North Africa (as well as in parts of Asia), this combination provides almost all the high-quality protein in the diet. And the cardiovascular-disease and cancer death rates for these regions are exceptionally low.[12]

Thus, complex carbohydrates in the form of whole grains, cereals, and legumes are an important part of traditional Mediterranean food. But food has to taste good for people to choose to eat it. And the use of olive oil in the preparation of these foods helps account for their widespread popularity. So we now turn to the discussion of the second component of the triad—the olive.

CHAPTER 5

The Olive

•

Dr. Scott Grundy is one of America's leading experts on diet and cardiovascular disease. He is the director of the University of Texas Human Nutrition Center in Dallas and a former chairman of the American Heart Association's Nutrition Committee. With both a medical degree and a Ph.D. in biochemistry, he is the quintessential medical-research "expert" on whom we rely for guidance about our health. Grundy is not an overly cautious medical bureaucrat. His research is innovative but scientifically meticulous, and he actively campaigns for increased public-health awareness.

Therefore, it was not surprising that Grundy received considerable publicity when one of his recent research projects was highlighted in the *New England Journal of Medicine.* [1] What caught the media's attention was the clear, unequivocal message he gave his interviewers. His recent clinical study, he explained, was based on a common-sense observation. In southern Italy and Greece, the traditional diet is high in olive oil, and people have a high daily total fat intake. But Greeks and southern Italians have low levels of plasma cholesterol, and their rates of coronary heart disease are also low. Olive oil, Grundy added, is a monounsaturated fat. So he decided to investigate the role of monounsaturated fats like olive oil in lowering blood cholesterol levels and offering protection from heart disease. And the results of that study, as published in the journal, support the concept that "a Mediterranean-type diet, high in monounsaturates, represents a reasonable alternative to a very low-fat diet for Americans."[2]

Some studies have shown that totally eliminating saturated fats in the diet and substituting small daily calorie totals of polyunsaturated fats such as corn oil have some dangerous side effects. The polyunsaturates seem to clean the system of both "bad" LDL cholesterol and also, unfortunately, of the HDL cholesterol vital for good health. In fact, some respected medical researchers have warned that a low-fat diet based solely on polyunsaturates increases the risk of certain cancers, due to the metabolic breakdown of polyunsaturates, which results in increased peroxidizing compounds known as free radicals.[3] "We may have been a little too rigid in our dietary recommendations," Grundy states, "saying that everybody has to eat the same diet to get the benefit of cholesterol lowering."[4]

So, seeking a moderate approach, Grundy and his colleagues set out to duplicate, under clinical conditions, the fat-consumption levels of the traditional Mediterranean diet and compare this "High-Mono" diet with diets high in saturated fats—"High-Sat"—and diets providing a low level of fat—"Low-Fat." They studied 11 men and 1 woman 49 to 69 years of age. The subjects were divided into three groups, each group following the three experimental diets for a four-week period during which the subjects were regularly tested for levels of blood cholesterol, LDLs, and HDLs.

Forty percent of the calories in the High-Sat and High-Mono diets were in the form of saturated, polyunsaturated, and monounsaturated fats, with either saturated coconut oil or monounsaturated olive oil making up more than half of this 40 percent. Carbohydrates made up an additional 43 percent of the calories of these two experimental diets. The Low-Fat diet contained only 20 percent of daily calories as fat, equally divided among saturated, polyunsaturated, and monounsaturated fats. The subjects' body weight was kept constant by adjusting total daily calories, and the subjects were not permitted any rigorous exercise during the three months of the study.

When the data were all compiled, the researchers discovered compelling evidence that the traditional Mediterranean diet offered protection from heart disease without increasing the risk of contracting those cancers associated with a high polyunsaturated-fat diet.

Compared to the High-Sat diet, the High-Mono diet, rich in olive oil, lowered total LDL-HDL cholesterol by 13 percent, while the Low-Fat diet reduced total blood cholesterol by only 8 percent. More important, the High-Mono diet reduced dangerous LDL cholesterol by 21 percent but did not reduce beneficial HDL cholesterol at all. In contrast, the Low-Fat diet "significantly reduced" HDL cholesterol and only reduced "bad" LDL cholesterol by 15 percent.[5]

The ratio between LDL cholesterol and HDL cholesterol was maintained at safe levels (more HDLs than LDLs) with the High-Mono diet, but, because of the decline of HDLs with the Low-Fat diet, the ratio stayed about equal.

In summary, it is probably safe to say that the low total blood cholesterol and favorable LDL-HDL ratios enjoyed by southern Italians and Greeks are attributable to the high proportion of both olive oil and carbohydrates in the traditional diet of these people. And it is interesting to note that these research findings parallel the results of the Crete-Corfu study.

"In the fight against heart disease," Grundy says, "olive oil may be a better weapon than the popular polyunsaturates like corn oil and safflower oil." For almost six thousand years, olive oil has provided the people of the Mediterranean Basin with their daily requirement of essential fats. And, as we have learned, olive oil continues to shield Mediterranean people from heart disease, even as they slowly adopt a more affluent diet. The important lesson here is that the monounsaturated fats in olive oil seem to sweep our circulatory system clean of dangerous LDL cholesterol while leaving our HDL cholesterol untouched.

Probably the most extensive survey to date of all aspects of the olive oil–health relationship was carried out by Italian medical researchers Publio Viola and Mirella Audisio. Their study, "Olive Oil and Health," which is being prepared for publication, offers dramatic evidence that olive oil is one of the most important elements in the traditional triad diet. Drawing on scores of studies by highly respected epidemiologists and biochemists, the researchers confirmed that inhabitants of those regions still following the traditional Mediterranean diet enjoyed overall better health than people who had adopted a more affluent diet. The role of olive oil in this pattern of healthful longevity transcended reduction of cardiovascular disease.[6]

Olive oil was also found to assist the natural rhythms of the digestive tract, reduce excess bile acids and tumor-provoking intestinal free radicals, and stimulate pancreatic secretion: all beneficial to digestion and proper metabolism.[7] In this regard, olive oil's role in preventing gastrointestinal diseases might parallel its importance in cardiovascular health. Further, the researchers discovered strong evidence that a diet rich in olive oil provides the best blend of mono- and polyunsaturated fats for infants who have been recently weaned from breast feeding. And even more interesting, the study summarized findings that clearly suggest that monounsaturated olive oil offers definite protection from the premature aging of tissue associated with metabolic peroxidation from excess free radicals. Diets too rich in polyunsaturates exacerbate this process, while the High-Mono pattern of the traditional triad diet inhibits this damage. This finding may help to account not only for the Mediterranean populace's good average longevity, but also for the excellent overall health so many Mediterraneans enjoy in their old age.

The authors of "Olive Oil and Health" compiled several independent studies that duplicate the results of the Crete-Corfu study. Clearly, olive oil's role in reducing serum LDL and preserving the proper HDL balance has gone beyond the theoretical to the scientifically factual. In the course of this research, Viola and Audisio also offered strong evidence that the health benefits of the traditional Mediterranean diet now rest on a solid foundation of scientific evidence. The traditional triad diet, they stressed, is characterized by moderation, especially in the consumption of those detrimental elements emphasized in more affluent diets. And the importance in the Mediterranean diet of cereals, fruits and vegetables, and fish plus the role played by olive oil form a uniquely beneficial combination.

Summarizing their findings on olive oil, Viola and Audisio offer this unqualified endorsement: "Owing to its balanced composition, olive oil has a protective effect upon the arteries, the stomach and the liver; it promotes growth during childhood and extends life expectancy, while at the same time its organoleptic characteristics produce a pleasing sensation to the palate." In other words, olive oil is good for your health, and it tastes great.

And we certainly agree with Viola and Audisio: the protective role of olive oil transcends its qualities as an effective cholesterol sweep and possible tumor inhibitor. In the traditional cooking of the Mediterranean, olive oil fills the same function as butter and other animal-fat shortening in northern European cooking and in American cooking. We all have a taste for rich, fatty foods; indeed, the words *creamy, buttery,* and *juicy* have become advertising synonyms for foods high in saturated fats. The U.S. Department of Agriculture's meat-grading system perpetuates this fat preference in our eating habits: prime beef is the top-graded beef not because it's the most nutritious, but because it has the highest fat content.

In this regard, Greeks and Italians are just like us. They demand their daily allotment of fat and complain when they are deprived. But they get their meal satisfaction from food prepared with olive oil, not saturated fat. This is important to remember when we consider replacing the unhealthy components of the affluent Western diet with the beneficial foods of the Mediterranean diet.

Olives provide more than just oil: as fruit, olives are also an important food in the Mediterranean. Moroccan and Spanish cooks prepare many rich, healthy seafood and vegetable dishes that include both green and ripe olives. Poor villagers use olives as a staple; and in some parts of North Africa and Greece, it is still common to see farmers making a meal of olives, bread, and a salad of cold boiled wild greens garnished with olive oil and garlic.

When we left the Foreign Service and moved to the Greek island of Rhodes in 1969, we ate the "normal" American diet that is heavy in meat and animal fats. During our last assignment in Tangier, Morocco, we had PX privileges at the U.S. Navy's Kenitra Base. Once a month we'd drive down the coast from Tangier and load up on American food at the base supermarket: frozen T-bone steaks, bacon, hot dogs, ground beef, butter, sour cream, and, of course, quart after quart of ice cream, not to mention gin, whiskey, and cases of stateside beer.

In our Greek island village of Lindos, however, we had none of these affluent luxuries. Greece was not yet a member of the Common Market; hard-currency reserves were low; and food imports were severely restricted. In short, we were given a forced, intense exposure to the Mediterranean village diet.

The first thing we discovered was olive oil. Lindos, like thousands of other Mediterranean villages, is surrounded by groves of silvery green olive trees. Every autumn, family groups pick up their long poles and trek into the hills for the olive harvest. Some of the gnarled trees, bent by the summer meltemi wind and the winter sirocco, are a thousand years old. And, even today with tourism's affluence, the villagers carefully tend each tree. They realize the wealth that resides in those twisted old trunks.

Soon after we moved into our whitewashed house, our neighbor, an elderly woman, offered us a hospitality present: a small soft-drink bottle filled with pale green-gold olive oil from that year's crop. This was probably our initial taste of truly good olive oil. It was delicate yet rich, smooth with an elusive, tangy aftertaste, almost like good wine.

Since there was no butcher shop in the village and we weren't enamored of canned meat (all that was available was fatty ersatz Spam from Czechoslovakia), we began to depend on local vegetable dishes, eggplant salad, lentils, broad beans, spinach, cold sliced beets, and so forth, slowly learning to combine the produce with increasing quantities of good olive oil and garlic. After having gone a few months through meat withdrawal symptoms, the symptoms had themselves withdrawn. We felt satisfied after each almost meatless meal, to which we added the odd (and some were very odd) chicken or canned Polish ham. Fish was available but surprisingly expensive because of the high demand from the tourist restaurants. And we soon developed a taste for Greek cheeses: creamy feta and rich mizithra, which, fortunately, was only available in the spring when the ewes had lambs. The Greek equivalent of Italian Parmesan, kefalotyri, added zest to many a vegetable dish.

In the process of changing our diet, we learned some important lessons. First, we discovered that olive oil is not "greasy," as many Americans believe. Even when we became fully "native" in our cooking, we found ourselves using relatively small quantities of the oil for dressing salads and vegetables because virgin olive oil was expensive in the village. And we learned to use a variety of "pure"-quality oil in hot dishes such as ratatouille, in baked goods, and for deep-frying. We discovered that olive oil was light and delicate enough for the dishes we were learning to love, especially the village salads that usually accompanied our dinner or that were the main component of our summer lunches. As our repertoire of recipes increased, we found a rich variety of tastes among the different types of olive oil.

The next important fact we learned about olive oil was that, ounce for ounce, it is no more fattening than margarine or butter. Again, good quality olive oil is so delicate and subtle that a small amount enriches a pasta or vegetable dish. And pasta became one of our staples, almost by default. Because the Dodecanese, of which Rhodes is the capital, had been an Italian protectorate after World War I, the local people had a taste for Italian as well Greek cooking. Good Italian hard cheeses were available locally, as was excellent Italian pasta.

We soon discovered that pasta could serve as the foundation for a great variety of satisfying dishes, as long as the pasta was treated well and olive oil was used in the sauces. Having both grown up on mushy, overcooked spaghetti and bland, garlic-free meatballs all smothered in thick tomato sauce, we were not prepared for *al dente* linguine primavera or rigatoni garnished with green onions (scallions) and garlic that had been delicately sautéed in olive oil.

But it didn't take us long to acquire a taste for such meals. By the end of our first year in Greece, we were living on a classic Mediterranean diet, probably receiving about 60 percent of our daily calories from complex carbohydrates and about 35 percent from olive oil. And we certainly didn't miss the heavy daily doses of butter, red meat, and dairy products. In fact, we experienced a reverse bout of culture shock when we returned to the States for a few months the following year. There wasn't much diet and health awareness in those days except among the people we would snidely refer to as "health-food nuts." We jumped back into the meat-and-potatoes routine with both feet. In the process, we made another discovery. Our system had become accustomed to a relatively meat-free—and, hence, animal-fat–free—diet, a diet high in monounsaturated oil, complex carbohydrates, vegetable fiber, and pectin. Slabs of fatty prime beef sat in our stomachs like . . . so much dead meat. Buttery sauces and gravies aggravated the situation. For our entire stay in the States that fall, one of us suffered from chronic heartburn bordering on gastritis, one became constipated, and we both felt bloated and dull.

In Greece, we had been averaging around 2,800 calories a day in the form of food that we could both easily and efficiently digest. Back in the land of burgers and milk shakes, we were eating about 3,500 calories a day, mostly in the form of "empty" calories and meat that was hard for our system to process. When we returned to Greece, we took up our adopted diet once more, and the digestive problems disappeared.

Years later we discovered that these digestive problems are potentially far more serious than many people realize. Gastric distress is an indicator of hyperacidity, and constipation while on a diet high in red meat (and with its dangerous metabolic detritus) can be a precursor to intestinal cancer. But necessity had led us to an inherently healthy diet that was also very palatable. This tasty, satisfying aspect of traditional Mediterranean food might seem a minor consideration to some scientists. However, it's a simple fact that people will not eat food they don't like. So the palatability of a diet is one of its most important attributes.

Seen in this light, the role of olive oil in the traditional triad diet of the Mediterranean takes on additional importance. It was olive oil in the form of dressings for vegetables and salads and as the basis of pasta sauces that had replaced the dangerous meat and dairy products that were so difficult for us to digest and metabolize. In the early 1970s, we had never heard of cholesterol or LDLs. But both our families had a history of heart disease, and we were concerned about our own future health. Over the years, we have maintained our taste for olive oil and pasta, for whole grains and a variety of green vegetables and legumes, for fish, and for wine.

Since many Americans are unfamiliar with olive oil, we should discuss the system used to grade the different types. In the past, hand presses were used to extract the oil from the crushed fruit, which was often placed in stacks of flat baskets and manpower applied to squeeze down a screw-type press. The first pressing in this process was classified as "virgin," "first pressing," or "cold-pressed." This classification system is still used today, although it no longer conforms to the methods of oil extraction. In the old system of hand pressing, the extraction of oil was often speeded up by pouring boiling water over the crushed olives.

But, in the past twenty or thirty years, powerful hydraulic and centrifugal presses have, for the most part, replaced the old-fashioned hand presses. The only time heat is applied in the pressing process is if the olive mill itself is not heated. Because of their general unfamiliarity with olive oil, however, many Americans still erroneously equate virgin olive oil with high-quality olive oil and dismiss the other main type of oil—"pure" oil—as a lower-grade, heat-extracted oil. This unfortunate comparison is often perpetuated by some of our leading food writers. Virgin oil has not needed to have impurities removed; pure oil has had impurities removed and has then been blended with a small amount of virgin oil to balance the flavor and aroma.

To set the often-confusing record straight, we quote here from the International Olive Oil Council's 1986 newsletter: "The grade or classification of the oil is determined by the oleic acid content of the oil and by standards of flavor, color and aroma. 'Pure' oils are those oils which have been refined to remove naturally occurring impurities; a variable amount of virgin oil is added to these 'pure' oils to enhance their flavors. More than 70 percent of the olive oil sold in the U.S. is graded 'pure.' Only 25 to 30 percent of olive oil is graded 'virgin' and 'extra virgin.' These oils must not have more than 1 percent (for extra virgin) or up to 3.3 percent (for virgin) acidity. Standards of flavor, color and aroma are higher for extra virgin than virgin oils."

Before we close our discussion of olive oil, let us compare the food value of a traditional American meat-and-potatoes dinner with a typical meatless Mediterranean dinner that features pasta and olive oil. We can attest that the Mediterranean meal is every bit as satisfying as the American dinner. And you be the judge of which is healthier.

The meal of pasta and olive oil is "healthier," as we have defined that term in this book. For example, the American meal has almost 25 percent more calories than the Mediterranean meal. And, equally important, the pasta–olive-oil dinner has only one-fifth the saturated fat of the meat-and-potatoes dinner. Less obvious, however, is the subjective satisfaction that the pasta meal offers. In the affluent West, a rich dessert such as pie à la mode is relatively common;

AMERICAN MEAL
(PORK CHOPS, MASHED POTATOES, GREEN BEANS, SALAD WITH DRESSING, ROLLS, APPLE PIE À LA MODE)

Item	Calories	Saturated fat (g)	Carbohydrates (g)	Protein (g)
2 fried pork chops	520	16	0	32
1 cup mashed potatoes (with milk and butter)	185	8	24	4
1 cup frozen green beans	30	0	10	2
Wedge of lettuce	12	0	0	1
2 tablespoons creamy dressing	130	2	4	0
1 white dinner roll	70	0	13	2
3 tablespoons additional butter (for potatoes and roll)	300	18	0	0
1 piece apple pie	350	4	51	3
1 scoop ice cream	255	8	28	6
Totals	1,852	56	130	50

people are not satisfied with a plateful of meat and potatoes, and they consume an additional 600 calories and 12 grams of saturated fat to achieve that satisfaction. Such a heavy dessert is unusual in traditional Mediterranean cooking. Certainly, ice cream and creamy confections exist in Greece, Italy, and Spain as well as in Turkey, Yugoslavia, and all of North Africa. But they are usually eaten as a holiday afternoon treat, a separate snack, not as a dessert course. Olive oil is so satisfyingly rich that heavy desserts simply are not appealing. In effect, the healthful combination of olive oil and complex carbohydrates in pasta protects Mediterranean people from the sweet tooth that plagues many Americans and northern Europeans. And, as we have seen, the obesity so prevalent in the affluent West has been relatively rare among Mediterranean people.

Now, let us turn to the third component of the Mediterranean triad diet—grapes and wine.

PASTA MEAL
(LINGUINE PRIMAVERA, FRUIT, WHITE WINE)

Item	Calories	Saturated fat (g)	Carbohydrates (g)	Protein (g)
2 cups pasta	400	2	74	14
2 ounces olive oil	485	6	0	0
½ onion	20	0	5	1
2 stalks broccoli	90	0	16	12
1 zucchini	30	0	7	2
1 carrot	20	0	5	1
Mixed greens	20	0	4	2
1 tablespoon olive-oil dressing	125	2	0	0
½ cantaloupe	60	0	14	1
2 4-ounce glasses wine	170	0	8	0
Totals	1,420	10	133	33

SOURCE: U.S. Department of Agriculture, Human Nutrition Center, Bulletin no. 72, rev. ed. (Washington, D.C., 1982).

CHAPTER 6

Grapes and Wine

The grape, *Vitis vinifera,* is one of mankind's oldest cultivated crops. Wine making has been going on for at least ten or twelve thousand years. In effect, Western civilization and the grape spread together as the Phoenicians, Greeks, and Romans colonized the rocky coasts of the "wine-dark sea."

By contrast, distilled spirits are a much more recent invention. The Western world was not introduced to grain alcohol or brandy until medieval times. And even then, Mediterranean peasants had neither the knowledge nor the resources to produce distilled liquor. As we've noted, the distillation process requires large quantities of fuel, a scarce commodity in the deforested Mediterranean. Furthermore, the elaborate metal plumbing and the understanding of chemistry needed to distill liquor were alien to the region's villages. So most Mediterranean people never developed a taste for hard liquor. Their traditional consumption of alcohol centered around moderate wine drinking with the midday and evening meals.

Given this historical pattern, Mediterranean people have been spared the health ravages engendered by widespread abuse of hard liquor.[1] Traditionally, a village clan grew its own grapes and made its own wine. An autumn's vintage had to be rationed throughout the year, and often a poor family had little more than the triad's three staples for their basic nutrition. For thousands of years up to the present, Mediterraneans have looked upon wine as a natural complement to meals. Anthelme Brillat-Savarin expressed this well in the nineteenth century: "A meal without wine is like a day without sunshine." It would be hard to find a more typically Mediterranean maxim.

Wine is the fermented juice of sound, ripe grapes. It is one of the most natural foods in our diets. In an age when much of what we eat and drink is the product of artificial processing and often dependent on omnibus—sometimes ominous—artificial flavoring, color, and preservatives for taste and shelf life, wine is a refreshing change. Although the wine-making process has been modernized and streamlined over the millennia, wine is basically the same now as it always has been.

Grapes ripen slowly through the spring and summer. The vine's leaves and grapes transform water, atmospheric carbon dioxide, and dissolved nutrients from the soil into sugars of varying complexity. Grapes also form acids while they ripen, along with hundreds of other "aromatic" components. When the grapes are ripe—usually by early autumn—the vintner tests the fruit for plumpness (moisture content), sweetness (sugar content), and acidity. Here, modern science can complement the age-old vintner's skill. But even the most high-tech vineyard in California still depends on the traditional human judgment of a master vintner for the proper timing of the harvest.

The grapes are harvested and crushed. The yeasts living on the grape skins are dissolved in the resulting juice, called "must." These "wine yeasts" of the *Saccharomyces* species make the vital process of fermentation possible. Over a period of a month or so, the yeasts in the fermenting batch of must convert the complex sugars into alcohol. Depending on the temperature and the sugar-acid ratio of the must, the fermentation process usually continues until the wine stabilizes at a mildly acidic level with an alcohol content of between 10 and 14 percent, with most good table wines averaging around 11 to 13 percent.

When this protowine is clarified (that is, the grape skins and other debris are removed) and is placed into either bottles or casks for consumption or further aging, respectively, it is basically organically stable. The fermentation process has been stopped because the alcohol has overcome the yeast culture. Bacterial spoilage is prevented by the combined alcohol and acid content. In other words, the wine is the refined essence of the grape, a natural food product that can last for decades (even a century or more) under the right conditions: a cool, dark, quiet storeroom (in other words, a wine cellar).

It was this attribute that made wine so important to the early imperial civilizations of the Mediterranean. When Greek city-states established colonies in Italy, France, and Spain, they also planted vineyards. The wine from these new lands became a vital commodity and was traded widely across the Mediterranean.[2] Indeed, by tracing the characteristic shape of wine amphorae found in ruins and shipwrecks, archaeologists can accurately trace the routes of ancient commerce. The Romans did things on a bigger scale than the Greeks; they transplanted Mediterranean vines to the Gironde estuary, the Rhineland, and the banks of the Loire. Only ten years after Columbus discovered the New World, Spanish missionaries were planting vine roots in the soil of Latin America. And the California vineyards—the linear descendants of the Romans' imperial outreach —took root more than two hundred years ago.

Given this fundamental position of wine in the taproots of Western civilization, it is not surprising that so much Judeo-Christian religious ritual involves wine. Nor is the ubiquitous role that wine plays in the Mediterranean diet surprising. For example, Italians currently drink approximately *10 times* as much wine as Americans —that is, per-capita wine consumption in Italy averages 24.2 gallons a year, compared with 2.4 gallons for Americans. But Italians have one of the lowest rates of alcoholism in the world. Indeed, the most traditionally Mediterranean countries—Greece, Italy, Spain, and Portugal—where low-alcohol table wine is traditionally consumed with meals, have the lowest rates of alcohol abuse and alcoholism in Europe.[3]

By contrast, northern civilizations, where distilled grain-alcohol liquors became popular in the past five centuries, have serious problems with alcoholism. When gin was introduced to late-seventeenth-century Britain, for example, the resulting social dislocation was devastating. On the frontier farms of colonial America, corn whiskey was the only practical cash crop. And socially corrosive alcoholism was rampant. As Thomas Jefferson remarked after returning to America from his long sojourn in France, "No nation is drunken where wine is cheap; and none sober, where the dearness of wine substitutes ardent spirits as the common beverage."

Jefferson was a keen social observer. Unfortunately, he did not have available the impressive body of recently assembled scientific evidence that proves that the benefits of moderate wine drinking go far beyond the prevention of alcoholism.

According to a report from the British Medical Research Council published in 1979 in the *Lancet,* there is a "very strong relationship between wine consumption and a low rate of death from heart disease."[4]

The researchers studied the death rates of 18 Western countries, including the United States. Two of these countries—Italy and France—are Mediterranean and had the highest per-capita wine consumption of the 18, and their death rates from heart disease were markedly lower than in the other countries. More important, there was a direct statistical correlation between wine consumption and reduced heart disease. The researchers found that in Finland and the United States, which had the lowest per-capita wine consumption, the adult-male death rate from heart disease was ten times that of France, where men drank an average of 2.5 4-ounce glasses of wine daily.[5]

Although the researchers did not unearth the mechanism that controls the apparent health value of wine drinking, they stated: "Wines are rich in aromatic compounds and other trace components which give them their distinct character—and it may be to these that we should look for the protective effect."

The researchers concluded that these trace components probably have a beneficial effect on the ratio of plasma HDL to plasma LDL and on blood-platelet formation (which is related to stroke). With dry British wit, the report's authors added, "If wine is ever found to contain a constituent protective against ischemic heart disease then we consider it almost a sacrilege that this constituent should be isolated. The medicine is already in a highly palatable form (as every connoisseur will confirm)."

This evidence closely parallels findings by leading American researchers. In 1980, the *American Journal of Medicine* published the

Honolulu heart study, which concluded that the rate of coronary heart disease decreases approximately 50 percent with moderate drinking. Moderate drinking is defined as the equivalent of 2 to 3 4-ounce glasses of wine per day.[6] By 1985, Dr. Ronald E. La Porte and his colleagues analyzed all the recent major studies on health and alcohol, and concluded: "Alcohol consumption is related to total mortality in a 'U' shaped manner, where moderate consumers have a reduced total mortality compared with total non-consumers and heavy consumers. Clearly, the results imply that moderate consumption, up to one to two drinks a day, is not detrimental and may in fact be beneficial for longevity."[7]

The Kaiser-Permanente Hospital Health Plan study published in *Annals of Internal Medicine* in 1981 provided much of the compelling evidence for the La Porte team's conclusions. This landmark study analyzed the health and drinking habits of 8,000 subjects over a 10-year period. Moderate drinkers (who drank up to 2 drinks a day) lived significantly longer and were 27 percent less likely to die from all causes than either abstainers or heavy drinkers (6 or more drinks per day). The dramatically increased longevity of moderate drinkers was shown to be due to much lower rates of heart disease, the Number 1 killer in the Western world.[8]

Slowly but steadily, Western researchers were establishing a body of data to explain the health benefits of moderate alcohol use as typified in the Mediterranean pattern of wine drinking with meals. But these researchers were justifiably cautious. Alcoholism is a scourge in many areas of the world, and it is unlikely that the medical research establishment will offer carte-blanche approval of all alcoholic drinks. For example, the British researchers were quick to point out that all alcohol consumption does not offer the same benefits as wine. In Scotland, where whiskey drinking is common—and hardly moderate—and wine drinking rare, the cardiovascular death rate is high.[9]

Moderate alcohol consumption, however, seems to offer protection from cardiovascular disease. Carlos A. Camargo and his associates at the Stanford Center for Research in Disease Prevention were among the first to identify the specific beneficial effects of such moderate drinking. As published in the *Journal of the American Medical Association* in 1985, the Stanford team concluded that a moderate drinker who consumes the equivalent of between 1 and 4 drinks (defined as containing 1 ounce of ethanol each) per day has a much higher level of serum HDL cholesterol. In particular, such moderate drinking increases the proportion of important HDL fractions, called apo A-I and apo A-II, to dangerous LDL cholesterol. These HDL fractions are widely believed to reduce the risk of cardiovascular disease.[10]

An editorial in the *New England Journal of Medicine* in 1984 seemed to summarize current expert opinion on the protective benefits of moderate alcohol consumption. "For a moderate drinker who has demonstrated the capacity to maintain intake at acceptable levels, there is no compelling reason to change that lifestyle and eliminate a pleasurable, possibly beneficial habit."

Clearly, then, moderation is the key to the health benefits of alcohol. And wine drinkers are among the most moderate consumers of alcohol. For example, wine drinkers in the culturally Mediterranean *départements* of southern France have a rate of alcoholism and cirrhosis only one-quarter that of their northern compatriots who traditionally consume "ardent spirits."[11] And in Italy, those provinces that have the lowest combined rates of heart disease and gastrointestinal cancer are in the south, where drinking wine with meals is a tradition established millennia ago and consumption of hard liquor is rare.

This different impact on health between moderate wine drinking and drinking hard liquor can be partially explained by the physiological and psychological effects of the two alcoholic drinks. Distilled spirits have been proven to cause the blood-alcohol level to rise up to 130 percent more than the equivalent amount of alcohol consumed in wine or beer. And peak blood-alcohol levels caused by ingesting hard liquor last longer. If, for example, a person consumes 2 whiskey or gin cocktails on an empty stomach, and another drinks 2 4-ounce glasses of white wine, the liquor drinker will not only reach a blood-alcohol level of 0.1 (legal drunkenness), but will remain above the so-called "threshold of impairment" for almost 2 hours. The wine drinker, however, will not reach drunkenness and will be only slightly impaired for less than 1 hour.

And we are talking about drinking on an empty stomach, a rarity among Mediterranean people. Almost universally, wine is served with food. When wine is consumed as a cocktail—mainly in urban centers—it is usually in the form of an apéritif like vermouth or Campari, and is almost always diluted with soda water. Among villagers, such drinks are uncommon. Mediterranean villagers like their wine; indeed, they drink it every day. But they tend to save it for mealtime.

This drinking pattern also allows wine to provide another important health benefit. It has been shown that wine aids digestion. Perhaps it is not an accident that Mediterranean people developed a taste for dry table wine that has an average pH level of 3.5 (the pH level of a domestic Chablis or Burgundy, for example), which is similar to our own gastric juices. Researchers have found that drinking wine with meals stimulates the secretion of gastrin, a vital digestive hormone.[12] Experiments in which solutions of 12-percent ethanol were substituted for wine showed no increase of beneficial digestive hormones. In addition to stimulating digestion, the soft, tangy bite of wine seems to increase our appetite. For this reason, over 50 percent of major metropolitan hospitals surveyed in a recent study reported serving wine with meals.[13] Since poor appetite in hospital patients can be problematic, American dietitians are now beginning to rely on one of mankind's oldest mealtime beverages: a glass of wine.

American nursing homes are also interested in using wine to stimulate appetite. In one study, nursing-home residents who received wine with meals were more socially interactive than those residents who did not receive wine with meals. Another group of elderly wine drinkers were reported to have a more positive outlook and were less likely to complain (that is, they were less depressed) than residents who did not drink wine. And in some homes, wine-drinking patients had improved blood pressure and slept better than those who were not given wine.[14]

None of this should come as a surprise. The relaxed, friendly social interaction for which the Mediterranean world is famous takes place almost entirely at meals, and those meals include table wine. In fact, what the recent American hospital and nursing-home research shows is that wine is a safe and an effective stress reducer when served with meals.

In light of the blood-alcohol comparisons cited above, this is readily understandable. Hard liquor gives the drinker a quick kick of ethanol intoxication followed by prolonged impairment. In effect, the pattern of the standard "two-martini lunch" is the rapid ingestion of about 4 to 6 ounces of pure ethanol (in the form of high-proof gin or vodka) on an empty stomach, which produces a sudden drunken glow. Although this intoxication breaks the stress of a difficult morning at the office, it also anesthetizes the gastric lining, reducing appetite and digestion. People who rely on hard liquor for stress relief may develop the symptoms of alcoholic malnutrition. When this pattern includes heavy tobacco smoking, the danger is greatly increased.

But in a typical Mediterranean meal, the preliminary "apéritif" period eschews hard liquor. Wine is served with small plates of appetizers—mézéthes in Greece, antipasti in Italy, and tapas in Spain. The stress-breaking qualities of slow alcohol absorption are maximized, while the sudden-"high" syndrome of hard liquor is eliminated. As we've seen, the wine stimulates appetite and digestion; and eating food, especially complex carbohydrates and olive oil, further moderates alcohol absorption. Typically, at a leisurely lunch or dinner, the wine drinking slowly keeps pace with the eating; there is no unnatural shock to the system like there is when one downs two martinis and follows the drinks with a slab of charred, fatty beef, buttered vegetables, and a cream-based dessert. The minimal stress relief obtained by this unhealthy affluent meal is more than offset by subsequent alcoholic depression (hangover) and indigestion.

Before ending our discussion, we should mention the benefits of grapes and raisins as fruit. Fresh grapes are an important source of food energy, dietary fiber, and vitamins and minerals during their two- or three-month summer and autumn seasons. When grapes are dried, their food value is not reduced. And raisins and currants do not need refrigeration and have an almost indefinite shelf life. They play an important role in the traditional triad cuisine of the region. Just as wine does, the complex carbohydrates of their natural sugars stimulate appetite as well as digestion. When served in rice and whole-grain dishes or plumped with other dried fruit to make a compote, raisins fill the desire for sweet food without resorting to the empty calories of refined sugar.

In Rome in October 1985, 500 scientists, researchers, and physicians gathered for the First International Conference on Food and Health. Wine drinking and health was the subject of lively discussions. The majority of the scientists supported the findings of the studies cited in this chapter: wine, taken in moderation especially with meals, protects us from heart disease, stimulates good digestion, and helps reduce the unhealthy stress endemic to modern urban life.[15]

The people of the Mediterranean Basin enjoy much better cardiovascular health than their northern European neighbors, have far less stress-related illnesses, and enjoy a glass or two of wine with their meals. And there is clear evidence that health-conscious Americans are increasingly following the Mediterranean example. Hard-liquor sales in the United States were down 6 percent in 1985, while wine sales are steadily rising. More than ever before, people who are interested in overall good health and fitness are turning to wine as their drink of preference, either as a cocktail or with meals. And these new wine drinkers are discovering what American connoisseurs have known for years: vineyards throughout the country offer us a wide variety of excellent wines. And given the high-quality of domestic wines available today, it seems that the typical Mediterranean pattern of moderate wine drinking with meals will soon become an American cultural tradition as well. When it does, we can expect to see the beneficial effects of wine drinking reflected in our national health statistics.

CHAPTER 7

Traditional Vegetables and Fruits

Just as we cannot live by bread alone, we also cannot live entirely on the three staple foods of the Mediterranean triad. For thousands of years, the region's inhabitants have supplemented their basic diet with the native vegetables and fruits that survive cool, rainy winters and long, dry summers.

As discussed in Chapter 1, Mediterranean kitchen gardens have been shaped by both harsh climate and sparse topsoil. The land is often steep and rocky, the surrounding hillsides overgrown with thorny maquis underbrush. Therefore, the vegetables must be hardy and have a good nutrition-to-volume ratio. Furthermore, these traditional vegetables have to have a long yield period throughout the year and a good shelf life without refrigeration.

The Neolithic revolution, during which agriculture was gradually developed throughout the world, began near the shores of the Mediterranean. People shifted from hunting and gathering to agriculture, retaining many of their earlier cultural habits such as culling wild food plants. All over the region, people still make use of the wild edible plants that flourish during the long, rainy winter and spring.

The Greeks call the goosefoots, thistles, and broadleafs that clothe the spring hillsides *horta,* or "greens." These dark-green, leafy vegetables have been an important source of food in the Mediterranean region since prehistoric times. Ironically, the steep, rocky hillsides that defy the plow provide some of the most nutritious elements of the diet. And it is probable that the hearty green vegetables in kitchen gardens originated from the wild native vegetation.

If we explore a typical Mediterranean kitchen garden, we will find broccoli, spinach, kale, beets, cabbage, and carrots, all of which have been grown in the region since classical times. Cauliflower, eggplant, and mustard greens are prevalent in the eastern Mediterranean but can be found throughout the area. Those vegetables from the New World—tomatoes and squash—have been fully assimilated into the cuisines, and no proper Mediterranean kitchen garden would be complete without them. The grape is the most ubiquitous fruit, but the fig is not far behind. Figs have a very ancient lineage, with references to commerce in the fresh and dried fruit dating to the oldest extant cuneiform tablets. The apricot, a native of China, probably found its way to the Mediterranean with Alexander's returning veterans. It was widely cultivated and has thrived ever since. Peaches and melons are also of ancient ancestry and can be found throughout the region.

When we try to summarize or typify the traditional vegetables and fruits of the Mediterranean diet, a pattern emerges: the oldest and most traditional of the plants fall into distinct families. Cabbage, broccoli, kale, cauliflower, mustard greens, and Brussels sprouts, for example, are members of the family *Brassicaceae;* their nutritional value is well established, but research has only recently discovered amazing additional health benefits of this class of vegetables. Spinach and its related wild dark-green cousins are nutritional clones and are biochemically very close to one another. And carrots and beets, which have been grown in the region since ancient times, are unique for their pigmented roots.

There is a common bond linking the members of the family *Brassicaceae* with spinach, carrots, and beets. Each of these vegetables is a rich source of vitamin A. Since the nineteenth century, the medical establishment has known that the vitamins in vegetables offer protection from scurvy and rickets. But only recently have researchers discovered that vegetables rich in vitamin A can protect us from certain cancers.

Vitamin A occurs in both animal and plant foods. In meat or milk, it is called retinol. The building blocks of vitamin A in vegetables are collectively known as beta-carotene. When we eat foods containing beta-carotene, our body releases beta-carotene's vitamin components. Vitamin A from both sources is fat-soluble—that is, our body can store a certain amount of this substance for use as a chemical catalyst during normal cell metabolism. But the beta-carotene found in dark-green and yellow fruits and vegetables fulfills another function: it is a potent antioxidant that actively combats carcinogens in our gastrointestinal tract, lungs, and reproductive organs.[1]

Repeated case-control studies in the past ten years, such as the Athens hospital research, have shown that those subjects (the "controls") who regularly ate dark-green and yellow vegetables and fruits —that is, the vegetables and fruits rich in beta-carotene—were less prone than others to contract the most prevalent (and life-threatening) cancers in the industrialized world: cancers of the lung, breast, larynx, esophagus, stomach, colon and rectum, prostate, and cervix. In these studies, the cancer victims (the "cases") irregularly consumed relatively small amounts of beta-carotene–rich vegetables and fruits. One group of researchers has postulated that beta-carotene derived from food sources somehow protects two groups of tissues in our body from the cancers to which they are most prone: the epithelial cells that line the lungs, gastrointestinal tract, and bladder; and the tissues of the breast, uterus and cervix, and prostate, which are sensitive to fluctuations of the endocrine system.[2]

However, artificial vitamin A—vitamin A in the form of a vitamin supplement—has not demonstrated the same protective qualities as naturally occurring vitamin A, although further research may show that these supplements are effective.

For the moment, though, the National Academy of Sciences–Nutritional Research Council has issued dietary guidelines based on an extensive review of recent scientific studies.[3] These guidelines urge Americans to increase their daily intake of fresh vegetables and fruits rich in beta-carotene. You will see from the following table that the list of recommended fruits and vegetables reads like a menu from a Greek-island taverna or southern-Italian trattoria.

Not only have researchers uncovered the protective qualities of beta-carotene, but they have also discovered the degree to which foods rich in beta-carotene seem to protect people from the most

	Serving	Vitamin A from beta-carotene (IUs)
Apricot (dried)	½ cup	7,085
Apricot (fresh)	1 average	960
Cantaloupe	¼ medium	3,400
Orange	1 average	290
Peach	1 average	1,300
Watermelon	1 average slice	3,540
Broccoli (cooked)	1 cup	3,800
Brussels sprouts (cooked)	1 cup	810
Carrots (cooked)	1 cup	15,750
Carrots (raw)	1 large	11,000
Peas (cooked)	1 cup	860
Spinach (cooked)	1 cup	14,580
Squash (winter)	1 cup	8,610
Tomato (raw)	1 medium	1,350

SOURCE: Based on U.S. Department of Agriculture, Human Nutrition Center, Bulletin no. 72, rev. ed. (Washington, D.C., 1982).

deadly forms of cancer. When Trichopoulou noted the "alarming" increase in the incidence of breast cancer among Greek women who had adopted the Western diet, she did not put this rate of incidence in perspective. Although cancer is, indeed, increasing at a rapid rate among those Greeks and Italians who have abandoned the traditional diet, the "Westernized" diet many have adopted still contains much less red meat and fat and more fresh beta-carotene–rich vegetables and fruits than the typical American diet. In fact, Greek women still have a low incidence of breast cancer, and Greek men —despite their high rate of cigarette smoking—still have a surprisingly low rate of lung cancer.[4]

One of the authors of the National Academy of Science's 1982 report *Diet, Nutrition, and Cancer* is Cornell University professor of nutritional biochemistry Dr. T. Colin Campbell. His partial explanation for public-health statistics such as those we see in Greece is as follows. Most cancers develop in a two-phase process. The first phase is the initiation or mutation of the DNA molecules in the nucleus of a single cell, usually by a carcinogen engendered by bad diet, such as the molecular "free radicals" associated with a high-red-meat, high-fat diet. This mutated cell may stay in the body for many years without turning into a cancerous tumor. The second phase, or tumor promotion, seems to be inhibited by substances such as beta-carotene (there are other substances found in some fruits and vegetables that have similar but less striking tumor-inhibiting qualities).[5]

This scientific observation is borne out in epidemiological studies. The age of a person when cancer occurs is extremely important. Thus, if we can modify our life style to delay or inhibit the active formation of cancerous tumors, we will have beaten the system to a certain vital degree. This may appear to be a brutally fatalistic statement, but every cancer specialist with whom we spoke validated it. They stress that cancer is not a major health problem per se, but that premature cancer that strikes men and women during their active years is an often unnecessary scourge.

Given this view of cancer and the mounting evidence for the dietary prevention or inhibition of tumor formation, let us examine the death rates for common cancers among certain matched age groups of men and women in Greece and the United States. This will give us a good indication of the overall incidence of these cancers and will provide a perspective on the protective qualities of the Mediterranean diet (see the table, below).

CANCER DEATH RATE PER 100,000 PEOPLE

	Age			
	25–34	35–44	45–54	55–64
LUNG CANCER				
Greek men	2.4	9.1	47.2	172.1
American men	0.8	11.8	76.2	213.2
COLON CANCER				
Greek men	0.3	1.7	4.5	11.8
American men	0.7	3.3	13.0	41.4
BREAST CANCER				
Greek women	3.6	17.3	35.3	55.0
American women	3.3	17.8	48.3	80.2

SOURCE: World Health Organization, *World Health Statistics Annual* (Geneva, 1984).

The statistics in the table become especially relevant when we recall that most medical experts consider these cancers to be directly related to diet (colon and breast cancer) or to smoking (lung cancer).

After discussing the statistics in the table with Greek researchers, we were able to collate some fascinating findings. Greek men smoke at least as much as American men, and the Greeks tend to smoke strong, unfiltered cigarettes. Furthermore, they have been smoking heavily for approximately as long as Americans—since the 1920s. Yet their death rate for premature lung cancer (between 35 and 54, according to experts) is one-third lower than that of their American counterparts. Researchers at the World Health Organization with whom we spoke tended to feel that a diet rich in beta-carotene might account for the favorable Greek lung-cancer statistics. These experts were quick to point out, however, that tobacco smoking was extremely detrimental to overall well-being and that no amount of dietary beta-carotene could effectively shield smokers from ill health.

When we consider the rates of premature colon-cancer deaths between the ages of 35 and 54, we see that the risk factor for American men is 3.3 times higher than for Greek men of the same age. The breast-cancer figures confirm the pattern: American women are almost 1.5 times as likely to develop breast cancer prematurely than Greek women in the same age group. Considering the fact that a large proportion of the Greek population still lives in rural areas where cancer detection and treatment is primitive by American standards, these statistics are even more impressive. Probably something in the Greeks' life style or environment is giving them a certain degree of protection from the deadliest forms of cancer plaguing the affluent West. And Trichopoulou believes that the relatively high proportion of traditional (beta-carotene–rich) vegetables and fruits in the Greek diet as well as the low amount of red meat provide the answer. Obviously, further research is needed and is, in fact, under way.

According to Campbell, the Greek researchers with whom we spoke are on the right track. "The relationship between diet and cancer, in my opinion, is now more persuasively established than the one between diet and heart disease."[6] Although beta-carotene–rich foods provide us with the natural vitamin A that can inhibit the cancer process, there is evidence, he adds, that the vitamin C found in citrus fruits, apricots, peaches, peppers, and tomatoes also offers cancer-inhibiting protection. Other researchers point to the members of the cabbage family as the source of yet another important group of compounds known as indoles, which have been proven by extensive case-control and clinical research to inhibit tumor formation.[7]

The high proportion of seed foods in the traditional Mediterranean diet might also partially account for the region's low rate of cancer. Researchers have shown that vegetables composed basically of edible seeds, such as beans, chickpeas, and cereal grains, contain a variety of compounds that inhibit tumor formation. And since the Mediterranean people have been eating edible seeds for millennia, we can begin to see the long pedigree of this healthy diet. For example, when British archaeologist Sir Arthur Evans unearthed the Minoan New Palace at Knossos, he found clay jars containing a variety of dried beans and lentils, which had been placed in storage about 3,500 years ago.

We must also consider the fiber content of these vegetables and fruits when we weigh their overall nutritional value. Vegetables such as eggplant, squash, broccoli, beets, and cauliflower have excellent fiber-to-calorie ratios; they are also high-volume foods that satisfy us and have no dangerous digestive end products. And when we examine peas, lentils, and beans, we find that their fiber content is even better than the above-mentioned vegetables and that their calorie-to-volume ratio is just as good.

The fiber found in the native citrus fruits, figs, apricots, and peaches is often overlooked. This fiber comes in the form of pectin, which is the natural thickening component of jams and jellies. According to Dr. James Cerda, director of Nutritional Laboratories at the Florida College of Medicine, however, pectin "is much different from any other fiber." The natural pectin fiber in fruits, he states, may be just as effective in lowering serum LDL cholesterol as many of the drugs now on the market.[8] Pectin fiber also speeds up digestion by giving bulk to stools.

All elements considered, the traditional Mediterranean diet may be one of the highest in natural food fibers in the world. And this, in turn, may account for the health and longevity of the region's inhabitants.

The cancer-inhibiting compounds such as beta-carotene, indoles, fiber, and vitamin C that abound in the fruits and vegetables of the

Mediterranean diet are no doubt of great importance. But the nutritional role that these foods play is perhaps just as important as their chemical make-up. In the triad diet, vegetables take the place of the meat and dairy products so favored in the affluent West; and fruits, both fresh and dried, replace the high-calorie, high-sugar desserts to which so many Americans and northern Europeans seem to have become addicted.

A vegetable stew such as ratatouille (or its myriad variants throughout the region) is a substantial dish, not a side course. The chunks of eggplant, squash, tomatoes, and peppers are sautéed with garlic and onions in olive oil, then slowly simmered to bring out their natural richness. When such a dish is served with pasta or crusty whole-grain bread, few people would hunger after red meat, fatty gravy, or a creamy dessert. As we shall see, these vegetable entrées are usually accompanied by small side portions of baked or broiled fish, beans, lentils, or chickpea spreads such as hummus. The entire meal contains ample fats, but basically in the form of monounsaturated olive oil. When fresh or dried fruit such as figs, apricots, peaches, or melon is served as dessert, the craving for sweets is answered in a healthful manner. The wine served with meals may also help meet the desire for something sweet. Furthermore, this typical Mediterranean village dinner is lower in calories than a meat-and-potatoes meal.

Many Americans will find the notion of a vegetable main course alien since we've been conditioned to believe that meat and dairy products are our best sources of protein and that we must consume high amounts of this protein every day to maintain good health. As we have seen, however, increasing scientific evidence is pointing in the other direction. And this same research is now presenting convincing evidence of the specific protective mechanisms that these foods can offer us.

Americans should find it relatively easy to increase the amount of desirable vegetables in their diet, while learning to cut back on the harmfully large portions of meat and animal fats. All across the country, restaurant salad bars now feature a variety of cruciferous vegetables, beans, and legumes that could be called a "Mediterranean smorgasbord." Later, dishes and meals that can wean us away from our heavy dependence on meat, dairy products, and refined sugar shall be considered. And, as we return to the more healthy nutritional patterns of our forebears, the transition will be easier because we will have learned how important these traditional foods are to our health and well-being.

CHAPTER 8

Fish and Fish Oil

Fish are an important and ancient food in the Mediterranean. The region is, after all, defined by the sea itself. And it was on the grapy-blue waters of the Mediterranean that human beings first learned to sail and fish.

British historian and diplomat Alan Davidson details this ancient fishery in his *Mediterranean Seafood*. He makes it clear that fish have been vital to the triad diet since prehistory. Davidson explains that the Mediterranean is really two seas: the western basin that is connected to the Atlantic by the Straits of Gibraltar; and the eastern basin that leads to the Black Sea and, since the 1800s, through the Suez Canal to the Red Sea and the Indian Ocean. Both basins are relatively shallow and warm, compared to the world's great oceans; and the sea's continental shelves are narrow. The high evaporation rate and paucity of feeder rivers (with the exception of the Nile, Ebro, and Rhône) has led to a high average salinity.[1]

All of these factors have had an impact on the fish of the Mediterranean and on the diet of those in the area who depend on seafood as a source of protein. The vast continental-shelf fisheries of the Atlantic and Pacific have provided plentiful cheap fish for centuries. But agriculture in northern Europe and North America has also offered competing bounty (especially in the twentieth century) in the form of cheap beef and pork. As we've seen, the raising of commercial livestock was never widespread in the arid and rocky Mediterranean region. However, fish were available. But fish bought at the market were expensive, and fish were difficult to catch in large numbers from the narrow coastal shelves of the mainland. Therefore, people learned to value fish as a luxurious yet vital component of their diet.

The fish on which Mediterranean people have traditionally depended fall into two main groups: (1) the shoals of immature schooling fish such as pilchards (sardines), anchovies, and mackerel; and (2) the large, deepwater swordfish and tuna, which are harvested by commercial fishermen. Salt cod is also a staple and was probably introduced during Roman times, fell out of favor in the Dark Ages, and was reintroduced in the nineteenth century.

Every Mediterranean village and town near the sea maintains a small fleet of open fishing boats in small harbors or drawn up on the pebbly beaches. And the colorful little scala is often the site of a seafood restaurant or taverna, as we saw in Chapter 1. In such establishments, one can observe the valued position of seafood in traditional Mediterranean cooking.

In North America and northern Europe, we usually treat inexpensive fish much the way we do cheap and bountiful meat. The fish is simply fried, broiled, or baked, and then remoistened with a creamy sauce or smothered in tartar sauce and served with a side order of potatoes and a boiled vegetable. We have grown used to the taste of butter-sautéed fish and thickly battered deep-fried fish. Indeed, as we've mentioned, some deep-fried fish fillets served in fast-food restaurants are cooked in beef tallow and contain more animal fat than a hamburger.

In the Mediterranean area, fish has never been cheap or bountiful, but generally it has been more available than red meat. Therefore, in the case of small fish, the entire fish is used, head and all. Fish soups such as bouillabaisse, stewed fish, fish-and-vegetable casseroles, and seafood pasta dishes are more prevalent than deep-fried fish. Almost all these dishes depend on an olive-oil base with lemon, garlic, and onion seasoning. Again, satisfaction level is achieved without resorting to animal fat or buttery sauces. The exception are fish such as red and gray mullet, which are grilled whole and dressed with olive oil and lemon. They are meant to be eaten with one's fingers, every morsel of the tender flesh picked from the bones. Fresh anchovies and sardines are usually sautéed in garlic-seasoned olive oil, then sprinkled with lemon juice, and eaten whole, bones included. Such seasonal dishes as tuna and swordfish steaks are often cooked with onions and fresh tomatoes, flavored with garlic and dill, and then baked inside oiled paper (to retain moisture). Variations of this dish range from the swordfish tagine of Morocco to the xiphias fourno of Greece. In the Mediterranean area, a meal featuring baked moist tuna or swordfish is considered a banquet. Fish is one of the few regular luxuries in Mediterranean villagers' lives; the people treat it with respect.

And the health benefits are substantial. Research completed in the past five years has proven that regular fish consumption, including the small portions found in the typical Mediterranean diet, can provide a shield against coronary heart disease and atherosclerosis.[2] Scientists have discovered that the oil of certain fish—especially swordfish, cod, salmon, tuna, mackerel, sardines, herring, and bluefish, to name a few, from the colder regions of the oceans— belongs to a special class of polyunsaturates containing omega-3 fatty acids. Research has shown that the omega-3 fatty acids found in some ocean fish have a profound impact on our ability to metabolize other fats. When eaten in small amounts on a regular basis, omega-3 fatty acids lower serum LDL cholesterol, particularly the very-low-density-lipoproteins (VLDLs), which are closely connected to coronary heart disease and atherosclerosis.[3] Researchers at the University of Oregon Medical Center in Portland have worked for years under Dr. William E. Connor, studying the effect of the omega-3s. According to Connor, 30 percent of Americans may have elevated levels of VLDLs. His team discovered that adding salmon oil to the diet could reduce total "bad" cholesterol levels by as much as 17 percent. And, equally important, the lipids in the omega-3s known as eicosapentaenoic acid (EPA) could control hormonal actions in the blood vessels that allow veins and arteries to dilate and to be swept free of platelets and cholesterol plaque.[4]

Compared to the omega-6 polyunsaturated fatty acids found in vegetable oils, the oil of fatty fish has been discovered to be up to *five times* more effective in sweeping the system clean of LDLs and

VLDLs. These important fish oils also have been shown to reduce other blood fats called triglycerides and to increase the amount of beneficial HDL cholesterol.[5]

All these findings on the benefits of fish and fish oil have received considerable attention in the world's medical journals. The *New England Journal of Medicine* recently featured two widely discussed research reports on this subject.[6] The best-known and most revealing epidemiological study was undertaken by the University of Leiden in Holland. Noting that Greenland Eskimos had low rates of heart disease and serum cholesterol despite their high intake of meat and fats, the Dutch researchers studied the relationship of fish to heart disease. In Zutphen, 852 men aged between 40 and 60 were followed over a twenty-year period. About 20 percent of the men ate no fish, while the other 80 percent regularly ate fish, often in small amounts. The fish eaters only averaged about 2 or fewer ounces a day. At the end of the twenty years, 79 men had died of coronary heart disease, and over four-fifths of these deaths occurred in the group that ate no fish.[7]

After completing a rigorous statistical analysis (which took into consideration such possible confounding factors as smoking, blood pressure, and weight), the Dutch researchers discovered that fish consumption was the most significant factor in distinguishing between those men free of heart disease and those men who had died from it. As little as 45 grams of fish a day—the equivalent of 1 or 2 fish dishes per week—seemed to offer this protection.

In terms of the traditional Mediterranean diet, Greeks currently eat a per-capita annual average of about 15 kilograms of fish, down from 16 kilograms twenty-five years ago.[8] This works out to an average daily fish consumption of 41 grams, very close to that of the healthy Dutch subjects. And this level of fish consumption is consistent with other countries in the region. In addition, Mediterranean people also regularly eat squid, octopus, and shellfish, although this seafood is less rich in omega-3 fatty acids than sardines, tuna, and mackerel.

We should mention the ancient ancestry of omega-3 fats in traditional Mediterranean cooking. For several thousand years, the people of the region have been preserving the oily essence of fish high in omega-3 fatty acids for use as a nutritional additive or supplement.

Throughout the Roman Empire, fish such as sardines, anchovies, or mackerel (or a mixture of these) were salt-fermented to produce a pale golden fish oil called "liquamen," which was used as a sauce for grain and vegetable dishes. It grew so popular that home fermentation was eventually replaced by liquamen factories in fishing ports such as Pompeii, Antibes, and Leptis Magna (Lebda) on the coast of North Africa. After the fall of Rome, this fish-oil commerce was disrupted, and people once more prepared their own fermented fish. The product changed over the centuries, losing much of its Roman refinement but retaining its omega-3 essence. By World War II, liquamen had evolved into salt-cured anchovies and sardines, and the product was no longer a clear golden liquid, but rather an oily block of preserved fish from which the cook simply gouged out a spoonful to flavor pasta or soups. Nevertheless, the cruder preserved fish contained just as much omega-3 fatty acids as the original Roman version.

Since the war, inexpensive canned fish such as tuna, sardines, mackerel, and anchovies, have become well established in even the most remote village. This canned fish is always packed in olive oil, so that the oil becomes the transfer vehicle for the omega-3 fatty acids. And Mediterranean people eat a lot of canned fish. When you visit any small village grocer in the Greek islands or Calabria, you will see the shelves bulging with brightly labeled canned sardines, tuna, and mackerel.

Clearly, then, seafood plays a beneficial part in the traditional Mediterranean diet. It should be relatively easy for Americans to take advantage of these benefits by replacing a portion of their dangerous foods with the healthy components of the triad diet. Currently, Americans are eating almost 150 pounds of red meat a year and less than 15 pounds of fish. In Japan—where the rates of cardiovascular disease are very low—many people eat six times that much fish.

But it is unlikely that millions of Americans will suddenly opt for the fish-heavy diet of the Japanese. Nor would such a cross-cultural transfer necessarily be a good idea; the Japanese suffer from high levels of diet-related stomach cancer as well as parasite disorders caused by eating raw fish. It is even less likely that people all across America will start chomping on raw seal blubber and chunks of raw fish, as do the Greenland Eskimos. Adopting the Mediterranean pattern of regular fish eating should not be hard, however. And, in a later chapter, we will suggest meals that take advantage of fish without resorting to buttery sauces or deep-frying in high-cholesterol tallow.

CHAPTER 9

Garlic and Onions

Characteristic of Mediterranean cooking is the use of garlic and onions. These two members of the lily family are eaten throughout the Mediterranean area. Read any Italian, Greek, Spanish, or Middle Eastern cookbook, and you will see garlic and onions listed among the basic ingredients in recipes ranging from the bouillabaisse of Provence through imam bayildi of Turkey to all sorts of appetizers, stews, and salads. The only meal during which onions and garlic are hardly ever consumed is breakfast, although many poor villagers still begin their day with a chunk of whole-grain bread dipped in olive oil and smeared with the pungent essence of crushed garlic.

Historic references to garlic and onions are numerous and of great antiquity. As early as 2000 B.C., Chinese herbalists praised the value of garlic. Ancient Sanskrit writings discuss both onions and garlic as important foods. And, according to the Greek historian Herodotus, those who built the Great Pyramids at Giza ate garlic and onions every day (with other Mediterranean foods such as radishes and lentils).

The health benefits of garlic and onions have long been recognized. Hippocrates found them to be an excellent aid to digestion and, in large doses, a beneficial laxative. Aristophanes held that garlic stimulated appetite and suggested that athletes and soldiers eat it regularly. And throughout more recent European history, philosophers and physicians have marveled at garlic's curative and protective qualities.

But most of the Western medical establishment has relegated the potential health benefits of garlic and onions to the realm of old wives' tales—until recently, that is. In the past decade, there has been an explosion of scientific research on the benefits of the two foods, and a mounting body of evidence suggests that our forebears were right all along.

We shall first examine the nature and benefits of garlic, then onions. Garlic's Latin name is *Allium sativum.* We eat the bulb of the plant, usually when it is dried, at the end of the growing season. Garlic and its close relatives—onions, shallots, and leeks—are all members of the lily family. The bulb is divided into a number of small, tight cloves, each of which is covered by a thin, paperlike membrane. When the bulb has been correctly dried, the cloves break easily away from the parent clump. In this state, garlic (or its relatives) gives off no pungent aromatic vapor. But when you cut, crush, or heat the dense, moist inner flesh of the bulb, the characteristic aroma of garlic is released.

This is the result of a surprisingly complex chemical reaction, which Western scientists have only recently traced. Garlic contains within its cells the amino acid alliin. When the cell walls are broken, an enzyme is released that converts the inert alliin into aromatic allicin, the central compound in garlic's distinctive flavor and aroma. All of the genus *Allium* (garlic, onions, leeks, and so forth) contain these alliin-allicin compounds to some degree—hence, their related eye-watering vapors and smell. Sulfurous compounds such as sulfides, disulfides, and trisulfides account to a large extent for this "burning" quality. In garlic, the most active sulfurous compound in allicin is diallyl disulfide.[1]

In the past decade, medical researchers around the world have been testing the age-old beliefs that garlic and onions somehow "cleanse" the bloodstream and promote general good health. And what they've discovered to date is astounding. In one highly publicized study reported in the *Tufts University Diet and Nutrition Letter,* Indian researchers at Tagore Medical College led by Dr. Arun Bordia gave a group of healthy volunteers the equivalent of 10 cloves of garlic a day, in the form of capsules of oil squeezed from fresh garlic.[2] The total blood cholesterol of the volunteers dropped by 14 percent, and their LDL cholesterol dropped by 17 percent. Equally important, the HDL cholesterol of the subjects rose by an amazing 41 percent.

In a similar study, Indian researchers gave volunteers a high daily dosage of crushed raw garlic.[3] At the end of one month, the subjects showed a substantial increase in serum compounds that inhibit blood-clot formation. Blood-clotting factors are important in the mechanism of atherosclerosis and stroke. It is believed that the blood of Westerners on a high-fat diet clots too readily, thus increasing the risk of heart attack or stroke.

In a continuation of the Tagore Medical College study, heart patients were divided into two groups: one received the garlic-oil–capsule treatment for eight months; the other did not. The results were even more convincing. The heart patients treated with high daily doses of garlic showed a marked decrease of LDL cholesterol and a significant increase of HDL.[4]

Similar research in Peshawar, Pakistan, has provided similar results. For seven days, subjects were fed a diet high in saturated fats. As predicted, their serum cholesterol shot up. Then the subjects were given the same diet with the addition of 40 grams of garlic a day. At the end of the second seven-day test period, the subjects' serum cholesterol had been significantly reduced, and a good LDL-HDL ratio had been restored.[5]

Extensive animal studies in the United States have duplicated the results of this pioneering Asian research. And long-range human-subject research on garlic's protective and therapeutic qualities is currently under way in this country.

An interesting study is being carried out by Dr. Myung Chi of the University of Nebraska at Lincoln.[6] Like the other researchers, he found that daily doses of garlic decreased subjects' LDL and increased their HDL. His evidence shows that the compounds in garlic inhibit those liver enzymes that metabolize saturated fats, thus permitting the dangerous fats to be eliminated from the digestive tract. And it does not matter if the garlic is fresh or not: "I've found that garlic—fresh, cooked or dried—can influence the way fats are metabolized."[7]

An exhaustive survey of this research, published in *Nutrition Research*, concludes that "the preponderance of research findings in both humans and test animals indicates the positive beneficial characteristics of garlic in lowering cholesterol and triglyceride levels.[8]

In 1979, Indian scientists discovered that regular consumption of garlic and onions by a large test group of subjects belonging to the Jain sect had a definite slowing effect on the subjects' blood-coagulation time, a major factor in preventing strokes.[9] A similar survey of non-Jains who did not eat garlic or onions showed a blood-clotting time closer to the Western norm. In America, researchers have tested a potent new anticlotting agent derived from garlic. Called ajoene (from the Spanish *ajo*, "garlic"), the compound could help prevent strokes, heart attacks, and hardening of the arteries. According to hematologist Dr. James L. Catalfamo of the New York State Department of Health, ajoene "appears to be more specific than aspirin, which should allow a more controlled therapy with fewer side effects."[10]

Turning to garlic's close cousin the onion, Drs. Katherine and Moses Attrep of East Texas State University have found that onions are a rich natural source of prostaglandin A-1, a hormone known to lower blood pressure. For the past five years in St. Elizabeth's Hospital in Brighton, Massachusetts, researchers have been studying the effects of onion extract on cardiovascular disease. Dr. Isabella Lipinska, director of the project's Lipid Research Laboratory, states that the findings have been positive. Although the subjects' total serum cholesterol has stayed about the same, there has been a significant increase in the proportion of HDL cholesterol (and a corresponding drop of LDL cholesterol) following daily doses of the extract equal to 1 to 2 onions.[11]

This research indicates that the allicin in both garlic and onions may contain the beneficial compounds. But the scientists all agree that it is too early to pinpoint the exact protective compounds in these foods. However, the volume and intensity of present research being conducted in this country on garlic and onions demonstrate that the American medical research establishment no longer considers talk about the benefits of these foods to be merely superstition.

And, finally, there has been some very promising animal research into the possible tumor-inhibiting qualities of garlic and onions. In one recent Texas study, a group of laboratory test animals was administered another of garlic's active compounds, diallyl sulfide, and was exposed to a known carcinogen. Another group was not given diallyl sulfide when exposed to the carcinogen. Those animals receiving the garlic chemical seemed to derive "significant" protection from carcinogen-induced cell mutation.[12]

In view of these findings, we may conclude that garlic and onions fulfill a nutritional function far beyond their role as food seasoning. But it is exactly this role—the zest they add to food—that gives them the opportunity to be used in greater amounts, thus increasing their potential health value. Although Mediterranean villagers who follow traditional eating patterns may not consume the equivalent of 10 cloves of garlic a day, they do eat both garlic and onions on a daily basis. Such people probably receive a regular protective dose of allicin in their daily diet.

In fact, Mediterranean cooks tend to start off almost every substantive savory dish by lightly suatéeing garlic and onions in olive oil. To this base can be added sliced tomatoes, which are then simmered until the tomatoes are tender and served with pasta, beans, and so forth. Or the basic garlic-onion foundation can be used to flavor such vegetables as broccoli or spinach, as well as the rich vegetable stews such as ratatouille. Soups often begin with this base instead of the meat stock favored in the affluent West. And when ground meat is included in such dishes as stuffed grape leaves, peppers, or cabbage, rice is added to the meat and this mixture is generously flavored with garlic and onions.

When we first went to live in Italy and Greece twenty years ago, friends in both countries would apologize for the lack of foreign restaurants. Italians (or Greeks), they would say, just like their own food; they're not tempted by fancy foreign dishes. What our friends were actually explaining was that traditional Mediterranean cooking was very good and satisfying. At that time people had not yet developed a hunger for the heavy meat and dairy products of northern Europe. Eventually, the Common Market worked its economic magic, and the questionable benefits of affluence spread across Europe. Although McDonald's and Wimpies have sprouted up in Milan and Rome, the Greeks have so far resisted this onslaught. But the persuasive powers of television advertising are making inroads even among the culturally conservative Greeks.

For the moment, however, the Mediterranean world has not abandoned its age-old attachment to garlic and onions. Tourists might exchange glances when they catch a strong scent of garlic from passengers on an overcrowded Rome bus. But these same suet-clogged northerners exude a definite lardy odor to Mediterraneans.

Ironically, it is this cultural chauvinism for one's own body scent that has prevented so many Americans and northern Europeans from adding garlic and onions to their diets. Overconsumption of raw garlic and onions can be a problem, but only for those who find the odor offensive. A normal daily level (1 onion and 2 cloves of garlic) of garlic and onions with one's meals, however, doesn't seem to produce socially unacceptable garlic odor. Americans should learn to be a little more tolerant. After all, what is worse—a little honest onion or garlic tang, or premature heart disease?

If you opt for heart disease rather than face social disfavor, you might consider several tested remedies for onion or garlic breath. First, and most important, remember that garlic is easily and quickly metabolized; that is one reason why it is such a good aid to digestion. Therefore, eat your garlic with dinner at home when you are not planning to go out. After your morning shower, the effects will have diminished. Another antidote to onion's and garlic's odor is to chew several sprigs of fresh parsley. If you're really sensitive to this scent, drink some lemon juice and water after your satisfying onion-and-garlic–based meal.

But we predict that you'll soon stop worrying about the smell of garlic and onions as you learn to appreciate their taste and health benefits.

PART III

Stress, Leisure, and Food

CHAPTER 10

Stress and Leisure

We spent our first winter in Italy living aboard a friend's boat in the Hannibal Marina, near Trieste in the industrial north. The huge Italcantiere shipyard was just across the channel from our pier, and on warm winter mornings we used to take our coffee break on deck, watching supertankers being assembled. But it was not simply this giant's Erector Set that held our interest. The workers at the shipyard were colorful and friendly, and they often grouped along the high concrete drydock to chat with us when we took the dinghy up the river into town on shopping trips.

After a few weeks, we began to notice certain consistent rhythms in the daily pace of the yard. The workday began promptly at 7:30, and for the next two hours the assembly buildings and yards were a bustling confusion of cranes, welding arcs, and clanging machinery. Then, at exactly 9:30, the siren sounded for the midmorning break. For half an hour, the workers relaxed, often grouped around food vendors' motorized carts, which offered coffee and traditional baked goods such as cannoli stuffed with nuts and dried fruit.

Two hours later, the lunch siren blew. The entire yard became silent; Italians take their lunch very seriously, and the Italcantiere shipyard scheduled a full hour and a half for this important ritual. Small teams of workers gathered at comfortable locations around the yard to share a meal. And the meals these men shared were not ham-and-cheese sandwiches on white bread. Every day, they began their lunch with either pasta or soup, served from large lunch pots brought from home. One man sliced generous chunks of whole-grain bread. There always seemed to be a boiled green vegetable of some kind—spinach, kale, or chard. On warm spring days, another man was given the task of making a salad of fresh greens, and we can attest from close scrutiny with binoculars that these salads were rich with raw onions and garlic. And every day, the men drank wine with their meal—not more than one or two glasses, but enough to add zest and help them relax from the pressures and tensions of the morning.

When the last of the salad dressing was sopped up with the last of the bread and the meal was over, the workers put away their pots and set about in earnest to enjoy the rest of their lunch break. Some curled up and slept in the shade, others quietly played cards, and still others took their wine glasses and assembled at the end of the dry dock to sing. The first time we witnessed this, we thought they were putting on a show for the benefit of the two *straniere* across the channel. Surely this was some elaborate hoax. But the foreman at the marina explained that impromptu choral singing was an old tradition among workers in the area. To us, however, it all seemed wildly exotic: welders and crane operators in rusty blue coveralls, grouped beneath the dinosaur skeletons of the tankers, raising their plastic wine glasses high as they sang arias from *Le Nozze di Figaro* or *Così fan tutte.*

At 1:30, the siren sounded once more, and the busy cacophony of shipbuilding resumed. Three and a half hours later, the workday was over. The men had been at the yard for nine and a half hours, but they had only worked for eight. Twice during the day, the pressures and stress of work had been broken: thirty minutes in the morning, and a full hour and a half at midday. Unlike factories in America or northern Europe, which give their workers a five-minute toilet break midmorning and a thirty-minute lunch break at noon, Italian plants almost all follow the pattern we observed at the shipyard. In addition, these companies all observe the traditional *fer' agosto,* in which the entire plant or office shuts down for the annual August vacation. In short, Italian workers (and their counterparts in Greece, Spain, and Portugal) work a forty-hour week eleven months a year, but they actually spend a longer time at the plant than workers in northern Europe and America.

The countries of southern Europe have certainly modernized their economies in the past twenty years, as the competition from Japan and from their Common Market partners have intensified; but the actual structure of the workday has not altered. A few years ago, for example, the Greek government tried to abolish the traditional four-hour summer midday break that had long prevailed in Athens. Stores, private offices, and even some government bureaus had been open from 8:00 A.M. until 12:00, closed from 12:00 until 4:00 P.M., and then open again in the cool afternoon from 4:00 P.M. until 8:00 P.M. The midday heat was spent over lunch at home followed by a nap, during which people put on their pajamas, shut the blinds against the sun, and went to bed.

This practice was so much a part of Athenian life that the government's efforts were to no avail. Within three months, the edict was reversed. Although government workers now put in a nontraditional straight shift from 7:00 A.M. to 3:00 P.M., with a very brief midmorning break, the large private sector still observes the split day with the long break. Such a staggered day allows people to relax over lunch and literally to sleep off the accumulated stress and tension of the busy morning. When they return to work at 4:00 P.M., it is as if they're beginning a new day.

This system works in cities such as Athens, Rome, and Madrid because they are basically devoid of suburban sprawl—that is, people own or rent apartments reasonably close to the city center, so their "commute" to work is relatively easy. But, unfortunately, this pattern is changing, and, along with it, the diet of the people. Some European sociologists, however, feel that it will be a long time before people in the Mediterranean give up their long lunch breaks and embrace the fast-food culture of America.

The fast food that has proliferated across the industrialized world is literally junk food. Although this food industry's lobbyists have been effective in pressuring government bureaucracies to lend their stamp of approval to the food products, we should not be taken in. Consider a double bacon cheeseburger on a white roll. What you have is about 500 grams of animal protein, saturated fats, and triglycerides. If the burger is flame-broiled, the level of protocarcinogens in it is increased; if it is fried in beef tallow, the cholesterol level shoots up. Add French fries cooked in beef tallow and a hydrogenated soy-milk "shake," and you have more saturated fat and carcinogens in one fast-food meal than you'll find in a month of Mediterranean village food.[1]

Now let's put this bizarre invention in its proper setting: crowded, brightly lit fast-food "outlets." These places are not designed for relaxation. They are designed by highly paid industrial psychologists to speed "customer flow." The colors, the bright lights, the smooth plastic, and the huge, prominently placed trash cans are carefully coordinated to make the customer eat, deposit his plastic detritus, and leave as quickly as possible.

Let us imagine that a harassed and tense person on a short lunch break arrives at the ordering counter and is handed his double bacon cheeseburger, small fries, and chocolate shake. Let us also suppose that he is alone (as millions are each lunch hour in our cities) and that his nerves are still jangling from the pressures of his morning's work. He is hungry, but the stress of the day has made his upper skeletal muscles and diaphragm tense. His schedule requires him to eat fast, but his body is hardly in shape to permit mastication and swallowing, let alone efficient digestion. Nevertheless, he gulps his half a pound of animal fats, sucks up the sugary, frozen hydrogenated soy oil, and scurries back to the office.

There has been almost no fiber in the meal and little in the way of complex carbohydrates to buffer the large slug of saturated fat. The person's liver and pancreas are confused by the biochemical information that this "normal" American lunch is transmitting from the predigestion zone of the near-spasmodic stomach. By the time the worker returns to his office, he is chewing an aluminum-based antacid to ward off "heartburn."

As the afternoon wears on, the sugar rush of the milkshake diminishes, and a sudden wave of fatigue grips him. So he combats this with two cups of strong black coffee.

He leaves the office at 5:00 and spends the next ninety minutes driving alone through rush-hour traffic. When he reaches his suburban destination, he greets his equally harassed wife (just returning from her job via the day-care center, where their children have been stored since school ended), and the family sits down to a meal of—you guessed it—fried pork chops, mashed potatoes, and so forth.

If this seems like an exaggerated description of an American office worker's day, ask yourself how many similar days *you* have experienced in the last year. And you should be aware that the type of day an average office worker must face may be healthier than that of his fellow worker on the factory assembly line or in the executive suite.

Having both worked in midwestern factories during college, we know what we're talking about. Sad to say, the stress on an automobile assembly line is even greater than in a modern office. If you make mistakes on the line, that line will eventually stop for the error to be corrected. Therefore, concentration is vital, even though the work itself is numbingly boring. The only way people can survive the assembly line is by working fast and intensely, and by not taking long breaks. Typically, lunch is twenty-five minutes—half an hour at the most. And many workers take their "lunch" at a bar across the street from the plant. There they relax with several shots of straight whiskey chased with beer. Almost as an afterthought, they may eat a quick sandwich of fatty lunch meat to slow the alcohol absorption in their stomach. When they get off at 3:30, they're almost sober and are becoming hungry again. They fight the traffic home and sit down at 6:00 to eat a dinner of fried pork chops . . .

And the executive? Lunch is business—there are clients to be *entertained* (whatever that means). In reality, lunch is often one of the most stressful parts of the day. There is usually a hierarchy of company authority at the table: senior executives are supposed to lead the invisible business being conducted, and junior executives are expected to offer assistance. The business at hand is hardly unstressful: a sale made or lost, an alliance forged or destroyed, a contract signed or ripped up. Executives do not stand at a Formica bar and swill boilermakers to break the tension of the morning on the line. They sit in leather booths and swill Chivas Regal, smiling tensely at the people across the table, making suitably neutral small talk. And at 6:00 or 7:00, they join the last of the rush-hour traffic, return home, drink some more hard liquor, talk to their children, then sit down to a meal of . . .

Exaggerated? Perhaps. But it is surely closer to the truth than many of us would care to admit. So what? you might say. America *is* high stress, but look at how efficient we are compared to the Italians and the Greeks. Those garlic-and-siesta countries are fun to visit, but they are hell to do business in. Maybe. But you can't "do business" without business people. In recent years, we've been losing around half a million people a year to coronary heart disease; paying the medical bills for CHD has cost us about $2 billion a year; and in 1985, American surgeons performed 160,000 coronary bypass operations.[2] Is that efficient?

The following table gives the per-100,000 CHD death rate for American, Italian, and Greek men between the ages of 35 and 64, according to the most recent World Health Organization data.[3] We have combined the WHO figures for acute myocardial infarctions (heart attack) and other ischemic heart diseases (including sudden cardiac death). Exhaustive research has linked both these heart disorders to diet and chronic stress, which we shall discuss in more detail below.

DEATH RATE OF MEN FROM CHD PER 100,000

	Age		
	35–44	*45–54*	*55–64*
America	47.7	217.8	579.9
Italy	26.8	125.9	324.6
Greece	32.8	99.9	262.3

You will observe that there isn't that big a difference among the three countries' CHD death rates for men aged 35 to 44, but there is a big gap in the 55-to-64 age bracket. These statistics would suggest a *chronic*, nationwide pathogenic (disease-causing) process at work in all three countries, but that this process is most severe in the United States. Conversely, there appears to be a beneficial process at work in Greece and Italy, with more benefits accruing to the Greek men. These combined processes seem to be most relevant in the group of men aged 45 to 54.

We would suggest (and there is a considerable body of scientific research to support us) that the combination of unhealthy diet, chronic stress, and lack of exercise of American men aged 45 to 54 might account for this wide difference in CHD death rates.[4] As we've seen, Greek and Italian men this age smoke more than American men do; so that factor is ruled out. But we know that high blood pressure and obesity (together with the factors mentioned above) play a major role in CHD deaths; so those two factors are probably at work. We also have seen that levels of serum cholesterol, especially LDL cholesterol and its dangerous subfactors such as VLDLs, are important components of CHD. But what about stress?

The average urban working American today most likely experiences more emotional stress than his Greek or Italian counterpart. Can this be proved scientifically? Probably, but we haven't found any research to support this premise. However, we have lived for extended periods in these countries, and, as trained reporters, we closely observe the world around us. And there is more stress built into the daily life of an American office employee or assembly-line worker commuting from the suburbs than into the life of his Greek or Italian counterpart. In the Mediterranean, the day is simply structured differently—a person has more time to relax, and people have developed stress-reducing habits to fill this leisure time. Unfortunately, as Mediterranean countries become more affluent, this pattern fades.

But what does one's emotional state have to do with coronary heart disease? Dr. Dean Ornish, in his *Stress, Diet, and Your Heart* (New York: Holt, Rinehart & Winston, 1982), maintains that chronic stress is one of the most pathogenic elements in the modern world.[5] Emotional stress—production pressure, rivalry, uncertainty, feelings of powerlessness, various threats (including that of nuclear annihilation), frustrations, and fears of failure and dismissal, all of which are endemic to modern life—provokes primitive physical responses collectively known as the "fight or flight" response. We all know this sensation—the adrenaline rush of anxiety, the thudding sensation of our heartbeat speeding up, the stiffening of our skeletal muscles and the tightening of our thorax, the dry mouth, the hot temples. What we do not feel, however, is the constricting of our arterial system, the microscopic clumping of blood platelets within these constricted arteries, and the increased blood pressure, which are an integral part of this response.

In primitive humans, this reaction to physical threat was a survival mechanism: constricted arteries with increased platelet aggregation bleed less; stiffened muscles absorb trauma better and turn limbs into better weapons. But in modern times, this response can be devastating since in most of the stressful situations of daily life we can neither fight nor flee. Instead, we slip across the street from the factory to the bar and down three boilermakers so that we might forget about that bastard foreman who's been riding us, or we anesthetize our spasmodic gut with a $5 expense-account martini while we smile across the starched linen tablecloth at the stubborn media director. But this does not help. The primitive adrenaline reaction to stress does not respond to sudden jolts of distilled liquor. The physical symptoms of fight or flight come from hormonal surges in the body: the hormone epinephrine, produced by the adrenal glands, causes much of the vascular constriction and blood-platelet clumping.[6] Alcohol alone will not counteract the effect of this hormone. And when we are under chronic daily stress, the atherosclerosis brought about by our high-saturated-fat, high-calorie diet becomes dangerous. Constricted coronary arteries become blocked by cholesterol plaque and then go into spasms. The result: acute myocardial infarction and other heart diseases.

Thus, to borrow from Ornish, the relationship between chronic stress and the dangerous diet of the affluent West becomes clear. Western diet lays the cholesterol trap in the cardiovascular system; chronic stress springs that trap by means of vascular spasm, platelet clumping, and hypertension.[7] And this deadly combination appears to be more than twice as common among American men aged 45 to 64 as it does among their Greek counterparts.

The "prophet" of stress-related diseases, Dr. Hans Selye of the University of Montreal, has been writing about the stress-CHD relationship for thirty years. He also believes that a variety of dangerous ailments, including cancer, may be related to chronic stress. More specifically, he theorizes that poor adaptation to chronic stress weakens the individual, so that the person is more susceptible to disease.[8]

These theories are fascinating, but there is nothing theoretical about the health statistics amassed in studies of chronically stressed workers. In one of the best known of these studies, cardiologist Dr.

Robert S. Elliot studied the rates of CHD among engineers and technicians at Cape Kennedy who were racing to put Apollo astronauts on the moon in 1969. The workers were under incredible production pressure: the stakes were high, yet the workers knew that their very success would signal a budgetary wind-down and the eventual elimination of their jobs. "In short," noted Elliot, "the project demanded an ever-increasing, if not frenzied, pace of production, with the ultimate reward of nearly inevitable dismissal."

These workers were very goal-oriented; they tended not to be emotional, but rather prided themselves on logical problem solving. Faced with the stress of a no-win situation, many became depressed. Alcohol abuse and divorce rates soared, as did heart disease. Sudden heart death—the form of CHD most clearly connected to stress— was 50 percent higher among young workers than their age peers employed elsewhere. And most of these fatal heart attacks occurred at the time of greatest stress—when layoffs were heaviest.

High-technology production pressures and job insecurity have become so widespread in today's economy that stress-related illnesses can be expected to increase. And all the experts we've read agree that it is imperative that people develop "coping strategies" which allow them to adapt to such chronic stress. In the next chapter, we shall explore ways to devise strategies that incorporate some of the lifesaving elements of the relaxed Mediterranean life style.

CHAPTER 11

Coping with Daily Stress

It would be foolish to assume that people in the Mediterranean Basin lead stress-free lives. In Italian, Spanish, and Greek cities, office and factory workers face the same kind of traffic, noise, congestion, and general unpleasantness experienced in New York or Chicago. Mediterranean villagers have worries about rain and drought, crop prices, interest rates, and all the other universal woes associated with farming. Yet, judging from WHO health statistics, people in the region seem better able to cope with stress than their counterparts in northern Europe or America.[1]

After years of living in Mediterranean countries and after interviewing European medical experts, we have concluded that, over time, people in the Mediterranean have developed coping strategies that work equally well in a village or an urban setting. However, we suspect that these stress-reducing patterns of daily life are not directly transferable to the urban (or especially the socially fractured suburban) precincts of the affluent West.[2] But at least we Westerners can emulate—even if we can't replicate—the coping strategies that have evolved in the Mediterranean region.

Since classical times, the extended family has been the basic social unit in the Mediterranean world. In villages and towns, the generations lived together under one roof, with an octogenarian grandmother often being an infant's nurse, while the child's mother worked the fields and vineyards. This basic extended family was joined by other, similar groups, producing a tightly allied clan. For better or worse, one never felt isolated; in fact, one never felt even physically alone. Problem sharing was *de rigueur,* and people voiced their hopes, fears, desires, and dislikes within the family circle on a daily basis. Holding back and being anxious alone was not considered normal among gregarious Mediterraneans. The concepts of privacy and individual initiative, which are so highly prized in America, were subjugated to the larger interests of family survival and group prosperity.

This family cohesion also prevailed when Mediterraneans, seeking work, moved to the industrial areas. Entire neighborhoods were settled by people from the same village, and several families would frequently share the same apartment. When Mediterraneans emigrated to northern Europe and America, they brought this pattern with them; and, to a certain degree, Greek, Italian, and Portuguese families in America have retained their cohesion through several generations.

The nuclear family, not the extended clan, is the basic social unit in contemporary America. Privacy and individual initiative—as well as individual responsibility—reign supreme. The majority of Americans today live in detached suburban houses that provide enough private sleeping space for a father and mother and two children. According to the 1980 Census, a majority of American families consists of two working parents who commute from the suburbs to their jobs (usually in two cars) and return home each night. What these statistics do not show is the physical and emotional condition of those commuters or the stressful daily pattern of their lives.

So, the first major social difference between the traditional Mediterranean world and the affluent West is the extended family versus the nuclear family. The second important difference is the pace of daily life. In the Mediterranean world, as we've seen, people tend to work eight hours a day, just as in America; but the actual daily period away from home is longer, due to longer meal breaks in factories or extended rest periods among shop and office workers. Also, given the urban geography in the Mediterranean, commutes to distant bedroom suburbs are almost unknown. A four-hour midday rest is, therefore, a practical alternative to the straight eight-hour day. And factory workers who leave the plant at 4:30 often sleep for an hour or two once they are home. This means that the evening meal is not usually eaten until at least 8:00 (in the winter) and even later during the long summer heat. In effect, the normal workday becomes two days, interrupted by either a midday rest or an after-work nap. This pattern is so important to the social fabric of the region that noise curfews prohibiting car horns, loud music, and even loud conversation are vigorously enforced from 1:00 P.M. until 5:00 P.M. in many Mediterranean towns and cities. It is interesting to note that, to a large degree, these coping strategies have evolved in response to the region's climate. Most Mediterranean countries endure a five-month hot season. Before the advent of air conditioning, shops and offices were unbearably stuffy at midday; and even today, the ubiquitous air conditioning of North America is less widespread in Rome and Athens than in Chicago and New York.

The slower, more relaxed pace of daily life has positive psychological effects and a definite impact on the role of meals in people's daily lives. Food is considered a source of sensual pleasure; a meal is seen as a relaxed, natural punctuation of the day, not as a pit stop for fuel. Fast-food outlets such as McDonald's have made inroads in a few Mediterranean cities, but these eateries are viewed as curiosities, not as serious institutions. The trattoria, tavolo caldo, or corner taverna, with oil-cloth–covered tables, wine casks, and an open kitchen, is common in the region. Here people can sit for an hour or more over a three-course meal rich in complex carbohydrates and olive oil, and accompanied by a glass of wine. Lunch is not only a relaxed celebration, but is also a respected institution. And the Greeks, Spanish, and Italians with whom we've discussed the subject all instinctively recognize the important stress-breaking function of meals.

We were amazed when, within the same week, two sophisticated Mediterraneans—one a Greek diplomat, the other a company director from Rome—independently offered their opinion that Americans seemed incapable of relaxing enough to enjoy a proper lunch. Don't people in America realize that it's important to break the tension of the day? they asked. They're beginning to, we replied lamely. But we knew that the majority of Americans viewed lunch as either a fuel stop or an opportunity to conduct business.

The traditional American pattern of eating the evening meal as soon as possible after returning home from work also puzzles many Mediterraneans. They consider it unhealthy to rush through the cooking and eating of a meal while one is still wound up tight with the stress of the day. What are Americans in such a hurry to *do?* we've been asked. We reached a depressing conclusion: most Americans rush through their stressful day and get their dinner eaten and the dishes washed by 7:00 P.M. so that they may use the next four hours to complete household chores and to watch television.

Even in these relatively liberated days, the responsibility of food preparation still primarily falls on the woman of the house. Therefore, a working woman has the additional stress of having to cook fast, even though she has not yet unwound from her hectic day. Supermoms who can "handle" this added stress may be in vogue, but many doctors feel that these women will pay the price by contracting premature cardiovascular disease.

In the Mediterranean, however, the stress of the day is broken at several points. Dinner, for instance, is a leisurely affair undertaken as a family activity *after* evening chores in the garden and school homework have been completed. Conversation, not television, provides the entertainment. This is a social occasion during which each family member rehashes his or her day and the stress of the outside world is vented and absorbed by the family as a group. There is a conscious savoring of the food and wine. And the attention paid to food provides a subtle benefit: if you are truly absorbed with the flavor and texture of rigatoni al pesto, it is unlikely that you will be reliving the tensions of a stress-filled day at the office.

Even though American society cannot suddenly transform itself into an idyllic Greek or Calabrian village, there are aspects of the relaxed Mediterranean life style we can emulate that will help us relieve the deadly stress of our hectic workdays. Those who feel that this stress is merely an acceptable irritant—the bill we must pay for our success—should once again compare the cardiovascular-disease death rates of Americans and Mediterraneans. Premature death is a terrible price to pay for prosperity; there is no success in an early grave.

With this in mind, let us have a look at ways Americans can better cope with pathogenic stress.

First, we are fairly well stuck with the nuclear family. Since it is highly unlikely that extended families or village-type clans will re-emerge in our civilization, we have to find alternative group interactions that help shield us from the impact of stress. As we proceed in this chapter, we will identify several such viable alternatives.

Second, American industry and commerce will probably never adopt the two-hour meal break or the four-hour rest pattern found in southern European factories and offices. But more flexible scheduling is possible in many workplaces, and managers are becoming increasingly aware of the cost of stress in terms of personnel losses.[3]

Third, we can learn to use our meals as more effective stress breaks and, while so doing, better integrate the benefits of the triad diet into our daily lives.

Let's begin with the morning and work our way through the day's schedule, suggesting stress-reduction techniques as we proceed.

Most Americans allow themselves just enough time at the start of the day to drive or take public transportation between home and the workplace. By so doing, they are beginning the day stressfully: they get caught in the morning rush hour and enter their shop or office with nerves jangling from the frustration of the unpleasant trip, their fight-or-flight responses pulsing along on an adrenaline high. Re-scheduling the traveling so that they can walk at least part of the way to work—preferably the final lap—and can thus arrive at the job site both physically and mentally relaxed provides a healthy alternative to morning stress.

We realize that this alternative might not be practical for every-one, but many of us could adapt. People in a car pool could be dropped off half a mile from the parking lot so that they could briskly walk for five or six minutes before work. Or they could get off the bus or subway a few stops before their destination and walk the rest of the way. Medical experts consider fast walking to be one of the most relaxing forms of exercise: it prevents stress by providing a natural outlet for the "flight" element of the stress response.[4]

Another alternative to the car, bus, or subway is the bicycle. Workers cycling to factories are a common sight in the Mediterra-nean world. The steady aerobic exercise of cycling is extremely healthful, and bikes rarely get stuck in rush-hour traffic. However, a densely congested city such as New York, with its kamikaze taxicabs and toxic street-level air pollution, does not offer a bicyclist a healthy alternative to public transportation. But Washington, Atlanta, Dallas, and other Sunbelt cities do provide well-conceived bicycle commuter paths.

You will be surprised at how different your workday begins if you learn to incorporate exercise into your daily transportation routine. And a brisk walk or bike ride at the *end* of the workday helps get rid of the accumulated stress of the afternoon.

About breakfast. Most nutritionists consider this to be our most important meal, yet many people either skip breakfast or eat junk food loaded with sugar and animal fats. Breakfast should provide at least one-third of our daily calories and is the ideal time to consume complex whole-grain carbohydrates and fructose-rich fresh or dried fruit. Also, we should learn to moderate our coffee and tea consumption and avoid refined sugar so that the stress we encounter during the day will not be exacerbated by a sugar-caffeine roller-coaster effect.

Throughout the business day, we should learn to take regular breaks, and these brief interludes should include some form of physical exercise. In the chapter notes, we've listed some books and studies on stress reduction. Almost all the authors agree that stretching, deep breathing, and brisk walking are excellent at relieving stress.[5] Some suggest meditation and yoga-like techniques. We have found that a ten-minute break every hour in which we stretch and walk about vigorously not only eases cramped muscles, but also helps clear the mind.

In this regard, all the experts we consulted repeatedly warn that the sugar-caffeine addiction institutionalized in the traditional coffee-and-sweet-roll break is a potent stress promoter, especially when this habit is aggravated by cigarette smoking. Therefore, we should consume fresh fruit juice and fruit instead of coffee and cheese Danish for our midmorning break. Fructose provides energy for our body without the stimulation and crash that we get from coffee and refined sugar.

Now, let's look at lunch. In the Mediterranean world, this is often the principal meal of the day, and it is followed by a rest. There's no better way to break the grip of stress than by taking a long, relaxed lunch followed by a couple of hours of sleep. Although this is not a practical alternative for Americans, we can adopt some of the elements of the Mediterranean lunch to suit our life style. First, we should always try to eat with other people, making lunch a social occasion whenever possible. And we should make it a rule to avoid shop talk during the meal. Second, if we eat in our office, we should disconnect our telephone—easily accomplished since the advent of modular units. Even though we might miss an important call, we will have gained valuable relaxation.

Let's consider choice of food. Ideally, nutritionists suggest, breakfast and lunch combined should provide two-thirds to three-quarters of our daily calories.[6] And, following the Mediterranean-triad pattern, these calories should be composed of 80-percent complex carbohydrates, vegetable protein, and monounsaturated fats such as olive oil. Therefore (as detailed in Chapters 12 and 13), foods such as pasta, vegetable soups, bean dishes, fish, and salads would be perfect for lunch, along with a glass of wine.

But should we eat pasta or whole-grain foods at every lunch? Italians and Greeks tend to eat such meals, and they live longer, healthier lives than non-Mediterraneans do, despite their less-developed health-care systems. In the Greek village, a large proportion of the complex carbohydrates is consumed in the form of whole-grain bread; in the Middle East, grain dishes made with bulgur, or cracked wheat, fill this role; and in the North African Maghreb, it is couscous—cracked wheat or millet—that plays this role. In Chapter 13, lunches are suggested that follow this pattern. We encourage everyone to learn to enjoy the more exotic carbohydrate dishes such as tabbouli and couscous, but we also include such standbys as macaroni salad and tuna casserole with shell pasta.

In terms of stress reduction, the advantage of such high-carbohydrate meals goes beyond the usable energy in the food; it also involves high-volume, low-calorie meal satisfaction. The "satiety" comes from a full stomach. When you look at an anatomical diagram of a human being, you can see that the stomach is close to the diaphragm, which becomes constricted during stress (the "knot in the stomach" is often a constricted diaphragm). And during stress, breathing is shallow and rapid, and the long skeletal muscles tense up. This is all part of the primitive fight-or-flight response.[7]

If you deposit 12 ounces of fatty beef and a pint of sugary frozen dairy substitute (the generic fast-food "shake") in your stomach when you are under stress, there is not enough volume to expand the stomach walls and help the diaphragm relax. You will probably get indigestion. That is, the gastric process will continue because fatty meat requires a long, complex digestion, but the stomach will be fighting against the rest of the system; and instead of relaxing during your meal, you will be under additional stress. The same holds true when you eat an expensive slab of prime rib after drinking two Bloody Marys.

A high-volume carbohydrate meal, however, aids relaxation by expanding the constricted abdominal cavity, thus restoring a relaxed breathing pattern. Once the breathing is relaxed, a sense of emotional well-being follows; and meal satiety leads to psychological contentment. The stress of the hectic day is broken.

In the final chapter, we suggest a week's worth of meals and a variety of substitutions. Although these meals will taste better and be slightly more nutritious if you take the time to prepare them from fresh ingredients, there are perfectly acceptable frozen and canned substitutes for many of the foods. We must add a word of caution here about canned foods. The American food industry has been very slow to reduce the high salt content of all canned foods, especially canned prepared dishes such as soups. Even some frozen foods have an unnecessarily high salt content. Salt has been proven to be a major culprit in hypertension. In a later chapter, we will suggest healthful flavoring alternatives to salt.

We strongly urge you to adopt the high-carbohydrate lunch as a consciously designed form of stress reduction. We also suggest that you form a lunch group of like-minded people at your workplace, and that group members take turns supplying the main course. In other words, Americans should learn to make lunch a relaxed group celebration, analogous to the meals we observed among the welders and shipwrights in northern Italy. When one of the group's members provides a dish such as minestrone or spaghetti con vongole, the others will probably show more interest in the food than they would in a dish of macaroni and cheese from the cafeteria steam table. And this interest in food, this focusing on the sensual pleasure of eating, provides yet another stress breaker. Since we cannot think about two things simultaneously, if we are absorbed in eating a colorful and spicy vegetable lasagne, we cannot be consciously preoccupied with an overdue report or balancing the quarterly financial statement.

And when you add a glass of good table wine to this lunch, the meal's stress-breaking value is increased—without the intoxication of a hard-liquor "fix." Many lunch counters these days sell good domestic wines in splits (6-ounce bottles), if a person wants wine with his or her lunch but has no one with whom to share it. But we suggest that you form a lunch group in which one person contributes the table wine each day. In recent years, the quality and variety of domestic wines have equaled—and have sometimes even surpassed —imported wines, and the price of domestic wines is often quite reasonable.

Let's assume that your group has a one-hour lunch break each day and that the meal takes forty-five minutes. In terms of stress breaking, a fifteen-minute head-on-the-desk snooze might be just the thing for certain people; for others, a brisk walk might be in order; still others might enjoy a hand of cards. What is important is that the relaxation of the meal be continued, albeit briefly, and that people do not put aside their fork and immediately hit the computer keyboard or make the first phone call of the afternoon.

Carrying this principle to the end of the workday, we suggest that the evening meal be consciously used as a stress-breaking interlude, not simply viewed as a biological necessity—the last of three fuel stops on the daily race course. Once more, we feel that the workday should be followed by some form of brisk exercise such as walking or cycling, which might be incorporated into the trip home. We also suggest that Americans, once home, stop dropping the briefcase and picking up the frying pan. If people are in such a hurry to eat dinner so that they can do a load of laundry and then vegetate before the television set, they are wasting one of the best parts of their day, and, in the process, they are again forcing food into their digestive tract before the body is relaxed enough to receive it properly.

The evening meal ought to be a group activity whenever possible, the supermoms surrendering some of their burden and sharing with the rest of the family the responsibility and pleasures of cooking. If you have children at home, they could placate their afterschool hunger with a snack (preferably fruit or whole-grain bread), then join their parents in the preparation of the evening meal. Supper does not have to be elaborate, but it should be tasty and varied. No matter how stressful your workday, you do have several hours of free time at home in the evening. And this free time can be pleasantly spent preparing poached fish provençale or chicken breasts and bulgur. The kitchen can become the warm, relaxed heart of the home (as it is in the Mediterranean region) as the family works together on the meal. The tensions of the day can be aired before you sit down to supper. Again, we suggest that you have some wine with your food and avoid the numbing effects of a hard-liquor cocktail hour.

The idea of involving the family in the preparation of the evening meal can work just as well with a group of friends. Similar to the lunch group, the dinner group can meet in different members' homes on successive days to prepare a common meal together. We first encountered this charming custom among an Italian film crew working on location in Morocco. Since we had a large house in Tangier with a well-equipped kitchen, our Italian friends assembled there several times after their day's shooting and cooked some memorable meals. As good as the food was, however, the relaxed atmosphere was even better. There is something about people cooking together— about the actual handling of food—that promotes relaxation.

We transferred this custom to America in later years. One of our favorite variations became the pasta party in which six to eight friends gathered to make fresh pasta, then took turns at the stove, each cooking a different sauce. An hour or two later, we were all ready to sit down and enjoy our creations, ranging from linguine primavera to cannelloni con funghi. And this pattern can work just as well for a baked fish or seafood dinner. The food is less important than the social exchange.

If you wish to expand such informal group dining, you could start a more formal weekend round-robin dinner club through your place of work or in your neighborhood. We joined such groups at several universities where one of us taught, and found them very enjoyable. The basic pattern of these groups is similar to the informal after-work gathering: members of the club meet at one another's home once or twice a month to prepare a communal meal for themselves which may have an ethnic theme. Thus, dinner one night might be Szechuan, another meal another night might be Greek, and so forth. Certain individuals or couples are responsible for certain courses;

others donate the appropriate wine; and everyone gets involved in setting the table and serving the food.

We know that many Americans will resist the patterns we suggest. In terms of health benefits, neither food nor wine has been taken seriously in our culture. However, this is changing as more people see the connection among nutritional habits, the pace of daily life, exercise, and overall good health.

In Chapters 12 and 13, we will discuss replacement meals based on the Mediterranean triad that you can incorporate into your life for good health and longevity.

CHAPTER 12

Adopting and Adapting the Triad Diet

From all the nutritional studies we have consulted, one common-sense maxim emerges: healthy food must not only be palatable, but it must also be familiar enough to bypass our cultural biases. For example, a ten year old in Barcelona will happily sit down to a lunch of calamares en su tinta (squid cooked in its own ink), and this meal will be extremely nutritious, especially when served with whole-grain bread and a tomato salad. But is it realistic to assume that an American child will come home from a Little League game and dig in to the same meal?

The corollary to this rule is equally important: healthful food must offer the same satisfaction as the unhealthy food it replaces. If you are going to eliminate a double bacon cheeseburger, French fries, and a chocolate milkshake, the replacement meal must offer the satiety elements of fats, red meat, and sweets *without* the high levels of saturated fats and refined sugars.

And an acceptable replacement diet must be practical and balanced. It is all well and good to suggest home-made minestrone—rich with lentils, beans, vegetables, and pasta—as a healthy alternative to the fast-food burger, fries, and shake. But how many working people have time to make soup from scratch? People eat fast food partially because they are under daily time constraints. And we must realize that the pressures brought about by having to accomplish a lot in a small amount of time will always be with us to a greater or lesser degree. Therefore, we are proposing a *modified* Mediterranean triad diet, tailored to meet the practical realities of contemporary Western life.

Much traditional Mediterranean cooking is relatively labor-intensive—lasagne and minestrone, for example. But we've discovered many shortcuts. Americans use microwaves, not brushwood beehive ovens, and nonstick pans, not copper pots; we often cook large batches and freeze portions for individual meals; we have plastic containers and plastic wrap, not tin lunch buckets; and the food processor has replaced the chopping block and the cabbage shredder. In short, American kitchen technology is marvelously adapted to preparing food quickly and efficiently. The premise of this book is that we all should be cooking *healthful* food using this technology.

Let it be noted here that we ourselves do not slavishly follow a transplanted replica of the traditional Mediterranean diet. We eat red meat, and we have been known to enjoy the occasional ice-cream cone on a warm summer evening. However, we have adopted the basic nutritional principles of the triad diet in our daily meals.

- We have cut our fat intake down to approximately 30 percent of our daily calories, and most of that fat is in the form of olive oil.
- Whole-grain foods and complex carbohydrates (including pasta) make up about half our daily calories.
- We drink moderate amounts of wine with our meals, and wine-based drinks such as Spritzers have replaced distilled spirits as evening cocktails.
- We flavor most of our main courses with garlic and onions.
- We eat fresh fruit and vegetables daily, especially those rich in beta-carotene.
- We eat ocean fish regularly, at least three times a week.
- When we do eat red meat, it is usually in small amounts, often used as a flavoring or minor ingredient in dishes such as lasagne.
- With the exception of hard cheese, we have eliminated whole-milk dairy products from our diet. But we do eat low-fat and no-fat yogurt regularly with fruit and use it as a base for sauces and dips.
- We have also eliminated most dishes in which refined sugar plays a major role.[1]
- Finally, we have drastically reduced the amount of salt in our diet by

eliminating most of the salt used in cooking. At the table, we have replaced salt with such condiments as freshly ground black pepper, oregano, and lemon juice.

But this is not a diet book per se. Nor is it simply a compilation of recipes. (A short bibliography of nutrition books that contain many recipes appears at the end of this book.) We offer instead a *nutritional pattern* that eliminates the dangers of the Western diet and incorporates the beneficial elements of the Mediterranean triad diet—that is, whole grains and complex carbohydrates, olive oil, and wine, as well as fruits and vegetables rich in beta-carotene, garlic and onions, and ocean fish. Often, the replacement dishes are directly transplanted from the traditional kitchens of the Mediterranean. Other dishes are modified to take advantage of American products and contemporary kitchen technology.

Now, some words about calorie consumption and that great American obsession, weight control. Any honest nutritionist will tell you that there is only one way to lose weight: eat fewer calories than you metabolize. There are two basic ways to achieve this goal:

1. Exercise regularly enough to burn more calories than you eat.
2. Eat fewer calories than your regular pattern of exercise metabolically burns.

Therefore, it is irrelevant to speak about one kind of cuisine or cultural diet being more or less "fattening" than another.

For the purposes of this book, we assume that you understand the basic principles of metabolism and obesity. We also assume that you, desiring longevity and health, will eat moderately and exercise regularly. So we have not assigned portion size or calorie values to the meals we describe below. The size of the portions will be up you. But we again want to stress a fundamental principle of the triad diet: high-volume, low-calorie carbohydrates offer greater meal satisfaction than low-volume, high-calorie meats. Remember this basic principle when you prepare your meals.

Before proceeding, we will explain certain principles and procedures of cooking with the key components of the Mediterranean triad diet. Many Americans are not familiar with olive oil, whole grains and pasta, or even garlic and onions. And relatively few Americans have discovered the zest that a dish takes on when wine is added to it. Vegetable dishes as a main course are little understood in this country, so we will offer some guidance in this important area. Finally, we will discuss the use of red meat or veal as a flavoring element, not a main ingredient.

Cooking with Olive Oil

As we explained earlier, all olive oils produced for sale in this country are "pure" in the sense that they have no additives and all impurities have been removed. The oils labeled "virgin" tend to vary in color and often have a more complex, full-bodied flavor than "pure" olive oils. There is such a variety of tastes among the many brands of olive oil that it would be wise to buy several kinds in small quantities, taste them, and decide which you prefer for salad dressings, which for sautéeing, which for deep-frying, and which for casseroles. Remember, olive oils are like wines in that their bouquet and taste depend on the soil and climate in which the fruit is grown. The current fad for "extra virgin" olive oil is all well and good, but experienced Mediterranean cooks prefer different grades of olive oil for different dishes. After some experimentation, you will learn which one to use when making salad dressing or mayonnaise, which when cooking with strong herbs and tomatoes, and which for a light wine sauce.

Color can be an indicator of flavor. The "greener" the olive oil, the more likely it is to have a very individual taste and aroma. But that doesn't necessarily mean that it will taste more of olives. Some pale olive oil is actually more flavorful than some green olive oil. Smell the oil. Different brands have different aromas. We keep several basic types on hand and try new varieties from time to time.

Olive oil stays fresh without refrigeration. Americans often make the mistake of refrigerating olive oil, and then they complain about the resulting coagulation. Store the oil in a cabinet, away from heat and light. Olive oil will last a few years if capped or corked. For economy, it can be bought in large tins, decanted into glass bottles, and then stoppered with a cork. Today, many supermarkets stock three or more brands of olive oil. You will find many more varieties in "gourmet" shops. Such stores even have olive-oil tastings from time to time to help you select the oil that is right for your needs and taste.

Olive oil may be more expensive than some other oils. But don't be tempted to dilute it with another oil. Part of the goodness of the olive oil is its purity, the lack of additives, and the variety of taste. And a small amount will go a long way. Our own attempt at economy is to buy large cans of the brand of olive oil we prefer. Italian, Greek, and Middle Eastern specialty stores abound in all large cities, and such stores charge reasonable prices for staples like olive oil.

Look for products packed in olive oil (tuna, artichoke hearts, and pimientos, for instance), and use that oil as part of the dish. But since olive oil is a fat, it should be used as sparingly as you would use butter, margarine, or any other fat. Your aim is to reduce total fat intake while substituting monounsaturated olive oil for saturated and polyunsaturated fats whenever possible.

In much French cooking, olive oil and butter are used together for sautéeing because butter burns easily and olive oil allows you to sauté food (to seal in the juices) at a higher temperature. We sometimes use a 2:1 ratio of olive oil and butter to quickly sauté veal scallops, which are then incorporated into an elegant main course; with this combination, you still get the rich taste of butter and have reduced the amount of saturated fats. Try combinations such as this when the flavor of butter is a must.

Again, because of olive oil's high burning point, it is excellent for deep-frying. The oil can be used over and over if it has not been overheated and has been strained between use. Also, olive oil that has been used for frying fish should be reused only for frying fish.

Olive oil can be used to make desserts, including cake (see Chapter 13).

As far as we know, no commercial mayonnaise uses olive oil exclusively. However, in today's American kitchen, there is almost always a blender or food processor available. There is no trick to making your own mayonnaise with this equipment. The instructions that come with the machine will give you the correct proportions of oil, vinegar or lemon juice, and egg. We use all olive oil, a combination of vinegar and lemon juice, dry mustard, a clove of garlic, just a touch of salt, and an egg. Kept covered in a glass jar in the refrigerator, this mayonnaise will last two to three weeks without spoiling. Make only small amounts (12 ounces) of mayonnaise at a time so that it can be used up before going bad.

One example of adapting the Mediterranean diet's nutritional benefits is our use of olive oil as a replacement for butter on popcorn. Since olive oil is an excellent vehicle for flavors, we sometimes gently heat a minced garlic clove or a pinch of red-pepper flakes in the olive oil, then pour it over our popcorn.

Cooking with Garlic and Onions

Garlic must be cut or crushed to release its active ingredient, allicin. But many cooks refuse to do this because the odor clings to the fingers. Rubbing a piece of lemon on your garlicky fingers should solve the problem. To combat garlic breath, chew parsley. In many Mediterranean recipes, chopped, fresh parsley is added—by the handful—to meat, pasta, and vegetable dishes that all begin by sautéeing garlic in olive oil.

Sautéed garlic and onions are the foundation of many Mediterranean dishes. First, finely chop 1 clove of garlic, and briefly sauté it over medium heat in 1 or 2 tablespoons of olive oil. Garlic burns easily and, once burned, becomes unpleasant-tasting, imparting this taste to the whole dish. If the garlic should burn, start the dish over again, using new ingredients. The next step is to add 1 cup of sliced or minced onions and to sauté them over moderate heat until they are golden. You can usually trust this process to timing and not have to hover over the pot. We use the microwave regularly for the basic sautéeing of garlic and onions in olive oil. (In a glass dish, pour 2 tablespoons of olive oil, add 1 chopped clove of garlic, microwave at high for 30 seconds, add 1 cup of sliced or minced onions, and microwave at high 1½ minutes longer. Stir the mixture, and proceed with the next step of the recipe.)

In some cases such as preparing a garlic-and-olive-oil sauce to accompany pasta, the garlic is only warmed in the oil, not cooked. Thus, the flavor is more intense.

Each culture's cuisine around the Mediterranean Basin has its own version of a garlic sauce to accompany fish or meat. In the recipes, we give two: Greek skordalia and French aïoli. In the eastern Mediterranean, whole cloves of garlic (bruised to impart their essence) are put in a bottle of vinegar to marinate. This "sauce" is placed on the table to be added to soup by each diner. Soups usually made from lentils, semolina, or even tripe are often eaten for breakfast on cold winter mornings.

Some recipes (for example, aïgo bouïdo—a Spanish soup made with a whole head of garlic—and the Provençal chicken cooked with 30 unpeeled cloves of garlic) call for huge amounts of garlic; but the garlic cloves are cooked a long time (1 to 2 hours) over low heat. The flavor is subtle; in fact, if you weren't told that you were eating garlic, you would never guess. And these dishes rarely cause "garlic breath."

There are many varieties and strains of garlic, ranging from elephant garlic—in which each head contains 8 to 10 very large cloves —to tiny, purplish heads. Rather than refrigerate it, keep garlic in a perforated ceramic holder (available in most kitchenware stores), away from the sun, and in a cool part of the kitchen. If you grow your own garlic, hang bunches by their long stems in a cool, dark place (the basement or garage) to dry, and use the garlic as needed. The flowering garlic plant is very pretty and is often seen growing wild on Mediterranean hillsides.

Dehydrated garlic in the form of flakes or powder lacks the active allicin desirable for good health and cannot be used successfully as a substitute for fresh garlic. Garlic cloves normally peel easily. An old trick is to bang the clove with the heel of your hand; the clove practically jumps out of its skin. And if you want to add a little garlic juice to a salad dressing, use a garlic press. But do not use the press for mincing; the garlic will pick up a metallic taste from the press.

Onions can add healthy gusto to almost any savory dish. There are dozens of varieties of onions, each of which has its uses: Bermudas are good for salads because of their sweetness; both yellow and white onions go well in any dish that has a long cooking time; green onions (scallions) need only the lightest sautéeing to impart their flavor and are sometimes used to garnish a dish. The texture and taste of onions change with the method of cooking. Try microwaving them whole —8 to 10 minutes on high; stand time, 5 minutes.

In order to peel onions easily, dip them in hot water to loosen the skin. To lessen the risk of teary eyes when cutting onions, peel them under running cold water, or place them in the refrigerator for a few hours before cutting them. Another trick is not to cut into the stem end of the onion (where most of the tear-producing cells seem to be) until the last minute. Today's food processors make the slicing and mincing of onions a less tearful task.

For "onion breath," chew parsley. Rinsing your mouth with lemon water also works. Or eat an orange or an apple after eating raw onions. Cooked onions leave almost no breath odor.

Cooking with Wine

Many people have not discovered the flavor-enhancing benefits even a small amount of wine can bring to food. The basic method of preparing a wine-enriched sauce for a meat, fish, or chicken dish is simple. After sautéeing the meat, fish, or chicken until it is done, remove it from the pan, raise the heat to high, pour in about ¼ cup of wine, and stir the liquid, scraping up the pan drippings. Let this mixture bubble a few minutes until the alcohol has boiled off and the sauce has been reduced to the desired consistency. Then pour the sauce over the reserved meat, fish, or chicken. Since all the alcohol is boiled off, there is no harm in serving children food cooked in this manner.

If we have an open bottle of red wine or plan to serve a cabernet or zinfandel with a meat dish, we'll use that wine in cooking; but white wine will do the trick just as well. In other words, cooking with wine does not necessarily mean preparing banquet food; wine adds gusto to everyday dishes, and you can use whatever wine you have open.

Another method of cooking with wine is to braise the ingredients in a mixture of water (or bouillon) and wine for an hour or more. The alcohol evaporates, and the wine adds its complex zest to the other ingredients.

The addition of "blush" wines (that is, white zinfandels, white cabernets) to our cooking repertoire has been a plus, since these wines impart more flavor to the food than white wine but are not as dominant as red wine. The creative cook can experiment without much risk of a catastrophe.

Fortified wines such as sherry, port, and vermouth will also enhance a dish, and they are much easier than wine to keep once they have been opened. But if you enjoy wine with your meals, as we do, it is not inconvenient to open a new bottle when you only need half a cup for a dish. The type of wine you have added to the food will be a natural choice to accompany the meal.

We frequently use wine for marinating. Most cooks develop their own favorite marinades over the years. We have two time-proven marinades: in the one for red meat, we combine red wine, olive oil, peppercorns, onions, garlic, and either rosemary for lamb, fennel for pork, or bay leaf for beef; in the one for chicken and fish, we mix together white or blush wine, olive oil, garlic, and fresh herbs (dill for fish is our favorite). Depending on the cut of meat, let it marinate in the refrigerator overnight or for a few hours (1 hour for fish). Barbecue or bake the meat, chicken, or fish, basting it with the marinade regularly, or prepare the dish some other way, using a bit of the marinade in a reduced sauce at the end of the cooking.

There are wonderful domestic champagnes on the market today. We suggest the following for a simple yet elegant dish: strawberries and champagne or, even better, raspberries and champagne. This light dessert is not only perfect on a warm summer evening, but provides a delicious finale to a special dinner.

Choosing which wine to use with what is a matter of personal taste. Basically, we stick to dry wines in classic combinations of red with meat and white with chicken and fish. However, a light red wine can just as easily enhance a poultry dish. The trend toward lighter food is probably matched by a preference for lighter, drier wines by Americans, not just at the table but in our cooking. A certain amount of experimentation will help develop a personal balance of flavors.

Assuming that you wish to follow the suggestions in this book for moderate wine drinking but are unfamiliar with wines, we suggest that you consult the manager at your local wine store. There are excellent, moderately priced domestic table wines. But there are also outstanding domestic vintage wines in all categories that compare favorably to their French and European counterparts; in many cases, the American wines outshine the European wines. The wine industry in America has come a long way. And as more and more Americans learn to appreciate good wine, they are discovering that vintage selections can be found right in their own back yard.

In the past few years, we have attended several American diplomatic receptions (in Italy, Morocco, and Greece) at which our embassy hosts served American wines. The sophisticated Romans, we noted, were especially enthusiastic about a Napa Valley Chardonnay. Indeed, some of our European friends report that California wines are considered an important addition to their own wine cellars.

Cooking with Pasta and Grains

Pasta comes in many shapes; choose the pasta for the type of sauce being served with it. The ability of the pasta to hold sauces is a function of its shape: for instance, tubular pasta such as rigatoni is best for thick, tomato-based sauces; thin, flat pasta such as linguine is readily coated with richer, more liquid oil- or wine-based sauces. More important than shape, look for pasta made from hard durum wheat (semolina). In many American stores, protein-enriched pasta is available under several brand names. It is higher in protein by about one-third and slightly lower in carbohydrates than regular pasta. And it compares well to the best-quality pasta we normally use. Homemade pasta is fun but time-consuming to make. Besides, due to the difficulty of making pasta in a home machine or by hand, most basic pasta recipes call for a combination of refined white flour and semolina. Pasta made from whole wheat, while more nutritious, has a different texture and taste, and takes some getting used to.

Most Americans' first experience with pasta is either spaghetti and meatballs with a heavy tomato sauce (usually more sauce and meat than pasta) or macaroni and cheese. These dishes taste good, but neither is good for you. The secret of a nutritious pasta dish is the sparing use of sauce. Almost anything can be used to make a sauce, but keep in mind those healthful foods that we have been talking about: olive oil, garlic, onions, green and yellow vegetables, fish, and wine. We are especially partial to vegetable-and-pasta combinations. Fish—even canned tuna and salmon—marry well with pasta shells or rotini. In a typical Mediterranean "meat-sauce" pasta dish, the actual amount of meat used is minuscule; it is there for taste and texture rather than as the major ingredient of the dish. (For instance, only ½ pound of lean beef or defatted sausage is used with 1 pound of fettuccine for four people.)

Chapter 13 will include several first-course, side-dish, and entrée pasta dishes, both hot and cold. Americans are "discovering" pasta and new ways to prepare it. And although there is a plethora of pasta recipes popping up in the food section of newspapers and in food magazines, we again suggest you experiment with these recipes, using the healthy foods of the Mediterranean.

Beyond pasta, there are other grains often used in the Mediterranean region. Couscous, from North Africa, is nutritious and easy to prepare. Look for it in the rice or pasta section of your supermarket. Bulgur, from Turkey, is, like couscous, a cracked-wheat product, easy to prepare, and good for you. We especially like tabbouli (a salad of bulgur, tomatoes, and parsley) in the summer (see p. 187). The only place corn meal is used in the Mediterranean area is in Italy, mostly in the north, in polenta. This dish is nutritious and tasty, whether it is served plain and hot, or cooled, cut into small squares, fried in olive oil, and sprinkled with Parmesan.

And then there is rice. From Spain to Greece and Turkey, white rice appears on the table as a main course (paella), a side dish (pilaf), in soups (avgolemono), and even as dessert (rice pudding). Although not as nutritious or as rich in fiber as whole wheat, it is still an excellent source of complex carbohydrates. To be sure you get the greatest health value, buy converted, enriched rice (the package should say "parboiled"). We have always followed the directions on the package with good results. But recently, while staying with our Turkish friends in Marmaris, we were served a wonderful plain rice dish. Every grain was separate and unbroken. It was explained to us that excellence in the culinary arts is judged not by how well the cook prepares imam bayildi or some other complicated dish, but on how tempting her rice is. Here is our friends' secret: soak 1 cup of converted rice in several cups of hot water. Let the water cool down, about an hour; pour off any excess liquid. Add 1 cup of cold water to the drained rice, bring the rice to a boil, and boil it uncovered for

5 minutes. Lower the heat to a simmer, cover the pot, and cook the rice for 25 minutes. Remove the pot from heat, uncover the pot, place a napkin over the rice, and re-cover the pot. Let the rice stand for about 40 minutes. (The napkin absorbs the steam.) Serve the rice with your main course, preferably one with a sauce that can be mixed with the rice. Or add a little warmed olive oil to the rice before serving the dish.

There seems to be a resurgence of local bakeries in America. While their baked goods like pies and sweet rolls are heavy in saturated fats and empty calories derived from sugar, these new bakeries also seem to be making goods for health-conscious Americans. Our own local bakery has whole-wheat bread on Fridays and Saturdays, which we can always freeze for use later on in the week.

And the smallest supermarket has a selection of breads rich in wheat or oat bran and whole grains. Pancake mix even comes in a whole-wheat variety and is good for you, if you can resist slathering it with butter and syrup (try low-fat or no-fat yogurt and fresh fruit). There are whole-wheat crackers and cereals. Many packages have the words "bran" and "fiber" emblazoned on the front. But read the list of ingredients carefully: "All Natural" doesn't preclude an overdose of sugar.

As we mentioned earlier, in the Mediterranean region, breakfast is often a nutritious soup. The most prevalent ingredient in this soup is usually some sort of grain or legume or combination of the two—semolina (farina) or lentil soup, for instance.

Cooking with Vegetables and Fruit

As nutritional research has repeatedly shown, most of us eat too few vegetables. This research also reveals why we must eat more vegetables: they are a natural source of essential vitamins such as beta-carotene and minerals such as calcium; and their fiber content is relatively high so that digestion is aided and LDL cholesterol is eliminated from the system before it can be absorbed.

Vitamin C is found in particularly large quantities in citrus fruit, tomatoes, peppers, and dark-green, leafy vegetables. These are all fruits and vegetables eaten almost daily in the Mediterranean region. The beta-carotene–rich vegetables and fruits (dark-green or yellow vegetables and fruits such as carrots, beets, broccoli, spinach, peaches, and apricots) are also plentiful in the Mediterranean diet.

A brief list of high-fiber vegetables that are extensively used in Mediterranean cooking would include beets, broccoli, cabbage, carrots, cauliflower, eggplant, kale, okra, onions, peppers, spinach, turnip and beet tops, and many wild greens like dandelion greens. Fruit plays a major dietary role in the Mediterranean region. Oranges, lemons, melons, grapes, apricots, and figs are eaten fresh in season. And it is common to see long trays of plums, apricots, grapes, and figs drying in the sun often on the flat roof of a village house.

The recipes will give more specific directions for cooking vegetables Mediterranean style. Many vegetables are eaten raw in salads. Others find their way into soups. But the most prevalent vegetable dishes are variations on vegetable stews such as ratatouille: the foundation of the dish—garlic and onions sautéed in olive oil—is prepared and is then followed by the addition of eggplant, peppers, zucchini or other squash, and lots of fresh tomatoes. Herbs are added according to region (in Greece, basil dominates; in Italy, oregano; in France, thyme; in Morocco, cinnamon or hot peppers).

The green tops of beets, turnips, and so forth are never discarded. They are rich in beta-carotene, vitamin C, and fiber, and, if cooked properly, they are very tasty (see p. 194 for method).

To conserve flavor and vital nutrients, cook fresh vegetables in very little water, or steam them. A pressure cooker or a microwave oven works well. We use these two pieces of kitchen equipment a lot, both for the sake of efficiency and because we like the results. Be careful not to overcook vegetables, whatever method you use.

We always make our own salad dressing. It takes only a minute and tastes much better than anything bought in the supermarket. Those little packets of flavoring have a lot of salt and sugar, and the taste is never as fresh your own dressing made with herbs snipped from the garden. We keep bunches of parsley, dill, coriander, and other herbs in season in a row of glasses containing an inch of water. Limp herbs brought home from the market will perk up within an hour. After a few days, snip the leaves of each of the herbs, place them loosely in individual glass bowls, and allow the herbs to dry in a dark cupboard. This only takes a day if it is not humid, and the results are excellent. If you buy or grow large amounts of herbs, it is best to use the standard drying method; wash and dry bunches tied at the root end; hang them upside down in a dark, cool place; and, when they are dry, snip the leaves and store them.

To make a basic salad dressing, pour 3 tablespoons of light olive oil into a 1-cup measuring cup, and add 1 to 2 tablespoons of red-wine vinegar (depending on the strength of the vinegar) or a combination of vinegar and lemon juice. Whisk the mixture to combine the ingredients. Add a pinch of dry mustard, a grind of pepper, a dash of salt if you must (we have weaned ourselves away from salt added to food in cooking), and fresh or dried herbs in whatever combination you have on hand. Whisk this mixture until it froths. Add about ½ clove of garlic, finely chopped. Don't toss the dressing with the salad until you are ready to serve, and then use the dressing sparingly.

Often in the Mediterranean, a salad is served undressed with fresh herbs strewn over it. Cruets of oil and vinegar are placed on the table. It's up to each person to pour oil (first) and vinegar in the proportions he or she likes. One of the great pleasures of eating a Greek salad of tomatoes, cucumbers, onions, olives, and feta sprinkled with oregano is mopping up the excess dressing with a piece off dense village bread. The dressing is rich with the essence of tomatoes and onions. To us and about 8 million Greeks, this dressing is far more delicious than butter on one's bread.

Cleaning and preparing fresh vegetables take more time than using frozen or canned ones, but it is worth the effort. If you eat frozen vegetables, do not overcook them, and buy them in their purest form—that is, with no sauce added. Canned vegetables are usually very salty, and their texture is much poorer than either fresh or frozen. If you must use them, simply rinse them and just heat them through.

When we first lived in Lindos, packaged snack food was unknown. So fruit and nuts filled this gastronomic niche. In our opinion, there is still no snack as delicious and healthful as a piece of fresh fruit. Since those rather idyllic days of our first years in Greece, prosperity has brought a plethora of potato chips and corn curls, "pizza" snacks

snapper, sardines, and eel. Squid is plentiful and is regularly served at the tables of both rich and poor. It is low in total fat but relatively rich in healthful omega-3 fatty acids, and can be used in a variety of dishes. Cuttlefish (sepia or inkfish) and octopus, which are also common fare in the Mediterranean, have similar nutritional value and deserve more attention in our cuisine. And, finally, shellfish should be reconsidered. After early concern based on miscalculations of their cholesterol content, shellfish have been restored to an important position in a healthy diet.[4] Thus, shrimp, lobster, prawns, and langoustes (saltwater crayfish) can once again be eaten in moderation without worry about cholesterol. These delicious seafoods, along with mussels, oysters, clams, and scallops, abound in the Mediterranean.

Choosing the right type of fish (cold-water ocean species) and shellfish will help the American cook prepare Mediterranean-type meals. Today, even in such inland cities as St. Louis, there is a regular supply of fresh seafood in the markets. Some fish freeze well (swordfish, shrimp, and squid) and also are available nearly everywhere in this country. Those people living on the East or West Coast have easier access to a large selection of seafood than those living in the middle of the country; they would do well to take advantage of this bounty.

Many cooks object to cleaning fish. Have the fish cleaned, boned, or filleted at the fish market; when fish is sold fresh at a supermarket, it is already prepared for cooking. Use it within a day of purchase. Or, if you must keep it an extra day, store it in the refrigerator in a tightly sealed plastic bag with another bag of crushed ice on top of it. Squid goes bad very quickly if not cooked within a day. Either use it on the same day you purchase it, or buy it frozen and keep it frozen until you are ready to cook it.

At some point, you will have to handle the fish you are going to cook, and that fishy smell will cling to your fingers. Have a cut lemon at hand, and counteract the odor by rubbing the lemon on your fingers as well as on any other surface with which the fish has come into contact.

The traditional Mediterranean methods of cooking fish are grilling the fish over charcoal (after having brushed them with olive oil and sprinkled them with herbs); poaching them in liquid, usually wine; baking them with other ingredients after having wrapped the fish in paper to protect the delicate flesh; and boiling them to make a hearty soup such as bouillabaisse. A modern method that we recommend is cooking fish in the microwave. (See the next chapter for recipes.)

Most of us are familiar with the methods used for cooking shrimp, lobster, mussels, and other seafood. But squid is "foreign." It is worth learning how to clean and prepare squid, for squid is both delicate in flavor and highly nutritious. First, cut off the tentacles, but do not discard them. Squeeze or cut the "beak" from the head, and cut the head from the body, just below the eyes. Now pull out the innards, including the pen or "cuttleshell," which is transluscent and flexible, and discard them. You can remove the outer skin by rubbing it off under running cold water. One recipe in this book uses the squid whole (stuffed), but in most of the recipes the squid is cut up into rings or pieces. Never overcook squid. Either quickly deep-fry it, or simmer it for an hour in a sauce; if the squid is treated any other way, you will wind up with rubber.

Cuttlefish has a stronger flavor than squid and is often cooked in its own ink. (The amount of ink in a squid is negligible.) Octopus, when cooked correctly, can be mistaken for lobster. Since, of the three, only squid is readily available in this country, we will not include recipes for either cuttlefish or octopus.

Cooking with Meat

American cattle and hog raisers have responded to consumers' increased health consciousness by breeding leaner beef and pork. And supermarkets are advertising these leaner cuts and are touting their rigorous trimming of fat. The taste of this meat has not been affected by the reduction of fat; it is similar to the grass-fed beef or lean pork of the Mediterranean. Most of that region's lamb, beef, and kid are naturally lean because there isn't the same rich grazing for the animals to fatten on as there is in the American West. And Mediterraneans have not yet discovered the cholesterol factories known in

America as feed lots, in which livestock convert grain carbohydrates to saturated fat.

Traditionally in the Mediterranean, unless an animal was young, it was tough. This led to meat being cooked in long-simmering stews or soups to tenderize it. Alternatively, tough meat was ground up, mixed with other ingredients, and added to a casserole.

Even then, meat made up only a small portion of the entire meal. By far, the greater bulk came from vegetables and complex carbohydrates. Although people in the Mediterranean region eat meat more often now than in the past, they still tend to eat small amounts of it. We have adopted this habit without any sense of sacrifice; we don't eat red meat more than twice a week and then only in very small portions. In fact, the idea of a large slab of steak on our plate (until a few years ago, our regular Saturday night feast) is repulsive to us.

Chicken is low in cholesterol, if you don't eat the skin; it is even better for you if you cook it after removing the skin. At the very least, you should remove all visible fat. Before the advent of frozen Common Market fowl, the Mediterranean chicken used to be a tough, scrawny creature that had served a life of egg laying and ended up in the pot. To make it tender, it had to be cooked a long time, which usually meant a stew of some sort. In other words, one bird mixed with vegetables and rice or pasta went a long way toward feeding a large family. Keep this principle in mind: for each diner, one piece of chicken such as a breast or a thigh, if properly seasoned and accompanied, makes an ample entrée.

Cooking with Dairy Products

We all need calcium for healthy bones. This is especially true for women, who are more prone than men to contract osteoporosis—the loss of bony tissue with age. Low-fat milk and dairy products are, therefore, vital. Some cheeses contain less saturated fats than others: feta, mozzarella (there is a skim-milk version), and Camembert. Plain low-fat yogurt is not only good to eat, but is also a nutritious substitute for sour cream. Many recipes calling for sour cream or crème fraîche will turn out just fine when low-fat or no-fat yogurt is used instead.

You will note in the next chapter that we do not feel that you must slavishly replicate in your home an authentic Mediterranean menu. In fact, there are aspects of the traditional Mediterranean diet you would do well to avoid (salt-cured fish and pickled vegetables are two that come to mind).

But we are convinced—as are research physicians and nutritionists in the World Health Organization and at leading universities in Europe and America—that the traditional Mediterranean triad diet comes close to attaining optimal nutrition. According to Dr. Jan Stjernsward, chief of the World Health Organization's Cancer Division, this diet offers us an excellent model. If the majority of people in the world's affluent countries would follow this pattern of eating, the diet would have "a *major* impact on reducing not only cancer but cardiovascular disease in the West. Such a diet would also promote general health and well being."[5]

CHAPTER 13

Mediterranean-Style Menus and Recipes

Here are some hints for adapting your eating habits to the Mediterranean diet:

- Use low-fat or no-fat yogurt and skim milk.
- Trim all fat from meat, and skin poultry before eating it.
- Leave peels on fruit and vegetables whenever possible.
- Use only small amounts of dressing or mayonnaise on salads.
- We suggest both juice and fruit for breakfast and another serving of fruit either at lunch or as a snack each day.
- When you take lunch to work, do not toss your salad with dressing until you are ready to eat it.
- Invest in an assortment of small plastic containers that seal securely.

M E N U S

MONDAY

BREAKFAST
Juice (preferably freshly squeezed citrus)
Whole-wheat toast with margarine or peanut butter
1 sliced peach mixed in ½ cup of low-fat or no-fat yogurt
Coffee or tea with skim milk

LUNCH
Salad of tomato, cucumber, onion, green pepper, and cabbage
    with olive-oil–vinegar dressing
2 pieces of "crisp" whole-wheat bread or toast with sardines
    or herring
Small bunch of grapes
6 ounces of white wine

DINNER
*Chicken and Bulgur
Fresh or frozen peas
Fruit sorbet
1 or 2 glasses (6 to 12 ounces) of California blush wine

TUESDAY

BREAKFAST
Juice (preferably freshly squeezed citrus)
½ grapefruit
"Bran" cereal with skim milk (choose a cereal with little
    or no sugar added)
Coffee or tea with skim milk

LUNCH
*Cold Tricolored Pasta Salad
Whole-wheat crackers
Thin slices of mozzarella
Apple
6 ounces of white or blush wine

*See the recipe in the next section.

DINNER
*Monkfish Medallions with *Skordalia
Potatoes boiled in their skin (use a pressure cooker)
*Beet Greens (or kale)
Carrot cake (purchased or homemade)
1 or 2 glasses (6 to 12 ounces) of California Sauvignon Blanc or
  Chenin Blanc

WEDNESDAY

BREAKFAST
Juice (preferably freshly squeezed citrus)
Half a small melon
2 pieces of whole-wheat toast with honey
Coffee or tea with skim milk

LUNCH
*White-Bean and Onion Salad
Rice-stuffed grape leaves (dolmádes) (from the delicatessen
  or canned)
1 sliced tomato and olives
Yogurt and fruit
6 ounces of Chablis

DINNER
*Veal Scallopine and Pasta with Wine-and-Mushroom Sauce
Steamed broccoli
Oatmeal cookies
1 or 2 glasses (6 to 12 ounces) of California Chardonnay

THURSDAY

BREAKFAST
Juice (preferably freshly squeezed citrus)
*Oatmeal and Plumped Dry Fruit
Coffee or tea with skim milk

LUNCH
*Salade Niçoise
2 pieces of "crisp" whole-wheat bread or toast
Rice pudding with raisins
6 ounces of white wine

*See the recipe in the next section.

DINNER
*Beans and Sausage Casserole
*Ratatouille
Fresh-fruit compote
1 or 2 glasses (6 to 12 ounces) of California red Zinfandel

FRIDAY

BREAKFAST
Juice (preferably freshly squeezed citrus)
1 whole-wheat English muffin or 2 whole-wheat toaster waffles
    (frozen) topped with yogurt and berries or honey
Coffee or tea with skim milk

LUNCH
*Chicken Salad in Pita Pockets
Coleslaw (cabbage and carrots)
Citrus-fruit salad
6 ounces of white or blush wine

DINNER
*Seafood Paella (Paella Marinera)
Green salad with artichokes and olives
*Semolina Pudding
1 or 2 glasses (6 to 12 ounces) of Chablis or Chenin Blanc

SATURDAY

BREAKFAST
Juice (preferably freshly squeezed citrus)
*Spanish Omelet (Pipérade)
Canadian or other type of lean bacon
Fresh fruit
Coffee or tea with skim milk

LUNCH
*Minestrone
Crusty bread
Any of the leftover desserts from the weekdays
6 ounces of red or white wine

*See the recipe in the next section.

DINNER
(an elegant meal suitable for guests or a special occasion)
*Meatless Borscht
*Salmon Steaks with Rotini and Julienned Vegetables
Salad of spinach and Bermuda onion rings with olive-oil–vinegar
   dressing
*Raspberries in Champagne
   1 or 2 glasses (6 to 12 ounces) of California Chardonnay with soup
   and salmon; champagne with dessert

SUNDAY

BRUNCH
*(suitable for a small or large group; all the dishes freeze well and can
reappear on the lunch menu during the week)*
Citrus juice and champagne (try the excellent champagnes
   of California)
*Warm Vegetable-Fettuccine Mold
*Seafood "Shells"
Rice-stuffed tomatoes and peppers
Homemade muffins or rolls (or good-quality ones from the bakery)
Melon halves filled with strawberries
*"Oil" Cake
   6 ounces of California champagne or Spritzers made of equal
   amounts of Chablis and soda

SUPPER
*Eggplant and Ground-Veal Casserole (Moussaka)
Salad
Baklava (store-bought)
California red Zinfandel or Cabernet

A WEEKEND BARBECUE

*Taramosalata
*Yogurt-Cucumber Dip
Crusty peasant bread
*Tabbouli
*Turkish-Style Beet Salad
*Swordfish Kebabs
Watermelon and cantaloupe
Oatmeal or bran cookies

*See the recipe in the next section.

A COCKTAIL BUFFET PARTY

(a meal consisting of the tapas of Spain, mézé of the Middle East and Greece, antipasti of Italy, and hors d'oeuvres of France)

COLD
Raw vegetables to dip in the sauces
*Taramosalata
*Hummus Turkish Style
*Eggplant Salad
*Yogurt-Cucumber Dip
*White-Bean and Onion Salad
*Turkish-Style Beet Salad
*Imam Bayildi
Stuffed grape leaves (dolmádes) (from the delicatessen or canned)
Marinated fish
Breads and crackers

HOT
Stuffed mushroom caps
*Vegetable Ravioli
*Meatballs Made with Bulgur
*Fried Squid Rings
*Jumbo Shrimp in Spicy Wine Sauce
*Bourekakia

Instead of serving spirits, offer several wines (Chablis, blush, white and red Zinfandel). Include fortified wines such as sherry, Campari, and vermouth, along with soda and juices to mix with them. Champagne is especially good at a party. Research has shown that the physiological and psychological effects of alcohol are proportionately less evident with champagne than spirits, beer, or even wine when the same amount of alcohol is imbibed.

*See the recipe in the next section.

R E C I P E S

The recipes that follow are mostly for those dishes mentioned in the previous text. Unless otherwise stated, quantities are for four people; however, it is very simple to halve a recipe, if there are only two people. When a recipe is labor-intensive, you may want to make a double batch and freeze half of it. Many working couples these days devote a few hours during the weekend preparing several meals in advance so that dinner during the week is relatively simple to put together. This takes organization and can only be done if you plan a menu before you shop for the week's food. Some people—ourselves included—don't like leftovers or eating the same food twice in one week. If you or members of your family feel that way, don't waste time preparing large amounts of food.

Many nutritious foods based on the Mediterranean triad are now being offered at take-out shops around the country. Such foods include a variety of pasta salads, dishes made with couscous or bulgur, and marinated shellfish or fish. If the name of the dish doesn't give enough information, inquire about the dish's ingredients.

When a recipe calls for ground veal, very lean beef may be substituted.

Most of the recipes do not mention salt. We use very little salt when we cook and suggest that, in accordance with the guidelines set forth by the American Heart Association, everyone try to reduce his or her salt consumption.

Appetizers

TARAMOSALATA

Both the Greeks and the Turks make a version of this fish-roe spread. The food processor makes short work of tedious hand chopping and the olive oil can be quickly incorporated into the spread using the same machine.

1 onion, peeled and quartered
1 clove garlic, peeled
Several sprigs parsley
1 cup tarama (salted fish roe, available in specialty
    food shops)
8 slices dry bread, soaked in water and squeezed dry
1 cup olive oil
3 lemons, juiced
Black olives for garnish
Lemon slices for garnish

1. In a food processor, chop the onion, garlic, and parsley. Add the tarama and bread, and process the mixture until it is smooth.
2. With the motor still running, slowly add to the mixture the olive oil and lemon juice, alternating between the two, and process this spread until it has the consistency of mayonnaise.
3. Place the spread in a bowl, and garnish the spread with the black olives and lemon slices. Serve this dish as a dip for vegetables or as a spread for crackers or crisp bread.

HUMMUS TURKISH STYLE ⚄

*Like so many dishes of the eastern Mediterranean and Middle
East, there is a lot of chopping and beating involved in the
preparation of this dish. But the food processor allows the modern
cook to accomplish in minutes what used to take half an hour.
Serve the hummus as a spread for crackers or bread.*

1 19-ounce can chickpeas, drained and rinsed
    (about 1½ cups drained)
¾ cup tahini (Middle Eastern ground–
    sesame-seed oil)
¾ cup fresh lemon juice
3 cloves garlic, peeled
Salt to taste
Paprika for garnish
Chopped parsley for garnish

1. Put the chickpeas in a food processor with the tahini, lemon
juice, garlic, and salt; process the mixture until it is smooth.
2. Transfer the paste into a serving dish, and garnish the hummus
with the paprika and parsley.

YOGURT-CUCUMBER DIP (TZATZIKI) ⚄

*This sauce or dip is good with fresh vegetables, crackers, fried
squid, or by itself.*

1 large cucumber
Salt
3 cloves garlic, peeled and minced
2 cups plain low-fat or no-fat yogurt
Fresh chopped mint leaves to taste (reserve some
    leaves for the garnish)

1. Peel, seed, and chop the cucumber. Place the cucumber in a colander, lightly sprinkle the vegetable with salt, and let the cucumber drain for 10 minutes. Pat the cucumber dry.

2. Mix together the cucumber, garlic, yogurt, and mint leaves.

3. Place the dip in a serving bowl, and garnish the dip with the reserved mint leaves.

BOUREKAKIA ✍

These Greek or Turkish savories make a great snack as well as a solid addition to a buffet dinner. And they freeze well uncooked.

CHEESE FILLING

½ pound feta
1 egg, beaten
½ cup chopped parsley, loosely packed

SPINACH FILLING

1 pound fresh spinach, rinsed well, dried, with
   tough stems removed
3 green onions (scallions)
3 tablespoons fresh chopped dill

8 sheets phyllo (may be purchased frozen in the
   supermarket)
Olive oil

1. Make the cheese filling by mashing the feta and combining the cheese thoroughly with the egg and parsley.

2. Make the spinach filling by chopping the spinach and onions (scallions), and cooking them in the microwave at high for 6 minutes. Remove the mixture from the microwave, and add 2 to 3 tablespoons of the cheese filling to the spinach mixture along with the dill. (Alternatively, cook the spinach and onions in ½ cup of water on

top of the stove until the spinach is tender, about 10 minutes. Drain the mixture thoroughly.)

3. Preheat the oven to 450°.

4. To make the bourekakia, cut each sheet of phyllo lengthwise into strips 2½ inches wide. Brush the top side of each strip with olive oil. Cover the strips with a damp cloth.

5. Working 1 strip at a time, place 1 teaspoon of filling at the bottom of the strip, and fold one corner of the strip diagonally over the filling, folding alternating sides and making a neat triangle. Put the triangle on a cookie sheet that has been brushed with olive oil. Repeat this procedure until all the filling and strips have been used up.

6. Brush the bourekakia with olive oil, and place the cookie sheet in the oven. Bake the bourekakia for about 15 minutes or until they are crisp and golden.

STUFFED MUSSELS ⚓

Mussels are very low in fat and cholesterol. Instead of serving mussels in the traditional manner—steamed open in wine—try this version from Bodrum, Turkey.

½ cup rice
40 mussels
3 onions, peeled and quartered
⅓ cup olive oil
1 tablespoon pine nuts
1 small tomato, diced
1 teaspoon ground allspice
Freshly ground pepper to taste
1 cup water
Lemon wedges for garnish

1. Cover the rice with hot water. Cool the rice, drain it, and set it aside.

2. Scrub the mussels, removing the beards.

3. In a food processor, finely chop the onions. Add them to a frying pan with the olive oil, and sauté them over medium heat for 15 minutes. Add the pine nuts and the reserved rice, and sauté the mixture, stirring it, for 10 minutes. Add the tomato, and cook the mixture 3 minutes more. Add the allspice, pepper, and water, and cook the mixture until the liquid is absorbed (about 15 minutes).

3. With a knife, pry open the mussel shells over a bowl, but do not separate the halves. Reserve the mussel liquid that has collected in the bowl. Lightly fill the shells with the rice mixture and press the mussels closed. Layer the mussels in a shallow saucepan, and add the reserved mussel liquid. Place a plate on top of the mussels to weigh them down during cooking.

4. Cover the pan, and cook the mussels over medium heat for 30 minutes. Simmer the mussels over very low heat for 30 minutes more. Remove the pan from the heat, and cool the mussels, keeping the saucepan covered. Clean the shells of the mussels with a paper towel as you arrange them on a platter. Garnish the platter with lemon wedges.

VEGETABLE RAVIOLI ⁄

This is our own version of a typical Italian dish. Instead of making pasta dough, we use won-ton wrappers as a shortcut. You may either steam these ravioli (see step 5) or fry them (see step 6).

½ cup finely chopped onion
2 cloves garlic, minced
1 tablespoon olive oil
1 cup trimmed, scrubbed, cooked, and puréed
  carrots
1 pound fresh spinach (tough stems removed),
  cooked and chopped
½ teaspoon freshly grated nutmeg *or* ½
  teaspoon hot red pepper flakes
1 1-pound package won-ton wrappers

1 egg beaten with 1 tablespoon water
1 cup tomato sauce *or* tomato wedges for
   garnish
Olive oil for frying

1. In a large frying pan, sauté the onion and garlic in the olive oil over medium heat until the vegetables are transparent. Remove the pan from the heat.

2. To the frying pan, add the carrots, spinach, and nutmeg or hot pepper flakes, and whisk the ingredients together until they form a paste.

3. Removing only 6 wrappers from the package of won-ton skins, place 1 teaspoon of this paste on one corner of each wrapper. Paint the edge of each wrapper—all four sides—with the beaten egg, and fold it over the filling into a triangle, pressing the edges of the wrapper together to seal the ravioli.

4. Place the 6 ravioli on a tray, and cover them with a dampened paper towel. Repeat this procedure until you have used up the filling. There will be approximately 4 dozen ravioli, depending on the amount of filling in each wrapper.

5. To steam the ravioli, place a single layer of filled wrappers at a time on the rack of a steamer. Put the rack over boiling water, cover the steamer, and steam the ravioli for 5 minutes, adjusting the timing, if necessary. Serve the ravioli with the tomato sauce (bottled or homemade) for a dip. Or you may serve them plain, garnished with tomato wedges.

6. To fry the ravioli, heat 1 inch of olive oil in a deep skillet to 375°. Place a layer of filled wrappers in the hot oil; make sure they do not touch each other. When the ravioli turn golden, they are done. Remove them from the oil with a slotted spoon, and drain them on paper towels. Repeat this step until all the ravioli have been cooked. When it has cooled down, the oil can be strained and kept for another use. Serve the ravioli hot without a sauce.

MEATBALLS MADE WITH BULGUR ⊀

These meatballs are lighter and better than when they are made with bread crumbs. They are good as part of a buffet or as the main course for a family meal.

¾ pound lean ground beef
½ cup uncooked bulgur
2 tablespoons minced onion
1 egg, beaten
Oregano to taste
Freshly ground pepper to taste
Olive oil
1 cup tomato juice (plus extra, if needed)

1. Mix the ground beef with the bulgur, onion, and egg. Season the mixture with the oregano and pepper. Form the mixture into walnut-sized balls.

2. Add enough olive oil to a large frying pan to lightly coat the bottom. Heat the oil over medium-high heat, and add the meatballs to the frying pan. After the meatballs have been browned on all sides, add the tomato juice, cover the pan, and simmer the meatballs for 45 minutes. Add more tomato juice or water if needed.

FRIED SQUID RINGS ⊀

The first time we had these at a reception in Morocco, we thought we were eating fried onion rings. Do not overcook the squid, or it will become tough.

2 pounds squid, cleaned (see p. 138 for the
    method)
½ cup flour
Olive oil
Lemon wedges
Yogurt-cucumber dip (see pp. 149–150 for the recipe)

1. Reserve the tentacles of the squid and cut the bodies in rings ½ inch wide. Dredge the squid in the flour, coating the squid lightly and shaking off any excess flour.

2. Pour olive oil in a deep skillet to a depth of ½ inch. Over medium-high heat, fry the squid in the olive oil until the squid are golden and tender. Drain the squid on paper towels.

3. Serve the squid with lemon wedges and the yogurt-cucumber dip.

JUMBO SHRIMP IN SPICY WINE SAUCE ⚹

Shrimp are found everywhere in the Mediterranean region. The following methods of cooking shrimp are easy and quick, and produce good results.

2 pounds shrimp, peeled and deveined
1 jalapeño pepper, chopped
Red-pepper flakes to taste
1 lemon, juiced
½ cup white wine
2 tablespoons olive oil

1. For microwaving, spread the shrimp in one layer in a microwave-safe dish. Sprinkle the shrimp with the jalapeño pepper and red-pepper flakes. Pour the lemon juice over the shrimp, and add the wine.

2. Cover the dish with plastic wrap, leaving one corner turned up for ventilation, and cook the shrimp at medium-high for 3 minutes. Stir the ingredients, and cook the shrimp for 1 more minute. Let the dish stand for 2 minutes. Continue with step 4.

3. If you do not use a microwave, in a frying pan sauté the shrimp in the olive oil for 1 minute, and sprinkle them with the jalapeño pepper and red-pepper flakes. Add the lemon juice and wine to the pan, and cook the shrimp, covered, over medium heat for 3 more minutes or until the shrimp turns pink. Continue with step 4.

4. Remove the shrimp from the dish or pan to a serving bowl.

Strain the sauce, and reduce it over high heat to ½ cup. Pour the sauce over the reserved shrimp. This dish may be served either hot or cold.

Soups

MINESTRONE

This recipe will serve eight. We put into the kettle whatever vegetables are on hand—from artichokes to zucchini. For a robust, nutritious winter meal, add diced leftover meat or lean ham.

1½ cups dried beans (a mixture of white,
   cranberry, and kidney beans)
2 onions, peeled and chopped
2 cloves garlic, peeled and minced
3 tablespoons olive oil
2 slices lean bacon, cut into small pieces
½ teaspoon dried basil
½ teaspoon dried marjoram
½ teaspoon dried thyme
4 tomatoes, seeded and chopped, *or* 1 small (14 ounce)
   can of tomatoes
1 cup red wine
6 cups water
1 cup diced carrots
2 cups mixed diced turnips, diced celery, and peas
⅔ cup small pasta (shells or stars)
8 tablespoons freshly grated Parmesan

1. Soak the dried beans overnight in water to cover. Drain the beans.

2. In a large kettle, sauté the onions and garlic in the olive oil. Add the bacon, basil, marjoram, and thyme, and cook the mixture for 5 minutes.

3. Add the tomatoes and wine. Bring the mixture to a boil. Add the drained beans and water,* and simmer the soup for 2 hours.

4. Add the carrots, and cook the soup for 15 minutes. Add the turnips, celery, and peas, and cook the soup until the vegetables are almost tender.

5. A few minutes before serving the soup, add to the kettle the pasta, and cook them for 5 minutes more or until they are tender.

6. Ladle the soup into individual bowls, and sprinkle 1 tablespoon of Parmesan on top of each serving.

*Before adding the water, you can microwave the mixture in a 4-quart microwave-safe casserole for 30 minutes at medium. Add 1 cup of water, the carrots, turnips, celery, and peas, and microwave the soup at high for 5 minutes, then at medium for 10 minutes. Pour the soup back into the kettle, add 5 cups of water, and bring the soup to a boil. Add the pasta, and finish cooking the soup.

LENTIL SOUP ⚔

This hardy, stick-to-the-ribs soup gets many a farmer through a chilly day. The addition of sausage or ham to the soup can turn it into a dinner entrée. If you decide to use sausage in this recipe, prick the sausage and cook it separately before adding it to the soup, making sure first to discard all the rendered fat.

1 cup lentils
6 cups water
1 onion, peeled and sliced
2 cloves garlic, peeled and chopped
1 carrot, finely chopped
¼ cup olive oil
1 bay leaf
1 cup diced ham *or* cooked sausage (optional)
Lemon wedges

1. Rinse the lentils. In a large pot, simmer the lentils with the water, onion, garlic, carrot, olive oil, and bay leaf for 1 hour (or use your pressure cooker or microwave, being sure to follow the manufacturer's instructions carefully). Discard the bay leaf.

2. You may serve the soup as is or purée it in a blender or food processor. Small pieces of cooked sausage or ham may be added to the cooked soup. The soup should be served with crusty bread and with lemon wedges on the side.

FARINA SOUP ✗

This is a bland soup that can easily be spiced up with a dash of Tabasco. It is, however, easy to make and nutritious.

3 tomatoes, chopped
3 tablespoons olive oil
⅓ cup farina
5 cups chicken stock (homemade or canned)
2 eggs
2 tablespoons milk

1. In a small saucepan, cook the tomatoes with a little water over medium-low heat for 20 minutes.

2. In a large saucepan, heat the olive oil, add the farina, and gently sauté the farina for a few minutes, constantly stirring. Add the tomatoes to the olive oil–farina mixture.

3. Add the chicken stock to the mixture, bring the mixture to a boil, lower the heat, and simmer the soup for 20 minutes.

4. Beat the eggs with the milk. Pour a small amount of the hot soup into the egg mixture, then transfer the egg mixture to the soup, constantly stirring the soup until it has thickened somewhat. Make sure the soup does not boil. Serve the soup immediately.

PASTA AND BEAN SOUP (PASTA E FAGIOLI)

This classic Italian soup is similar to minestrone but is thicker and richer-tasting.

½ onion, peeled
1 carrot
1 stalk celery with leaves
¼ cup olive oil
2 pork ribs *or* 1 ham bone
2 tomatoes, chopped
1 cup dried white or cranberry beans, soaked
    overnight and cooked, *or* 1 20-ounce can
    beans, drained and rinsed
3 cups beef stock (preferably homemade)
⅔ cup small pasta (shells *or* stars)

1. In a food processor, chop the onion, carrot, and celery.
2. Heat the olive oil in a large saucepan, and add the chopped vegetables plus the pork ribs or ham bone. Sauté the mixture for 10 minutes.
3. Add the tomatoes, and cook the mixture for another 10 minutes or until the tomatoes give up their juices.
4. Add the beans to the mixture.
5. Add the beef stock to the sauce-and-bean mixture, and bring the soup to a boil.
6. Add more water to the soup, if necessary.
7. A few minutes before serving the soup, add the pasta, and cook it until it is done. Serve the soup immediately.

MEATLESS BORSCHT ✍

This bright-red soup makes a dramatic first course. The slightly sweet flavor is especially refreshing in the summer.

4 beets, trimmed and scrubbed, with 2 inches
   of stalk
1 clove garlic, peeled
¼ peeled onion
1 cup chicken stock (preferably homemade),
   degreased
Low-fat or no-fat yogurt
2 green onions (scallions), thinly sliced, for
   garnish

   1. Cook the beets in a pressure cooker for 15 minutes, or cook them in a saucepan in water to cover for 45 minutes or until they are tender. Remove the beets from the pressure cooker or saucepan, straining and reserving ½ cup of the cooking liquid. Peel the beets when they are cool enough to handle.

   2. Cut the beets in quarters, and put them in a blender or food processor with the reserved cooking juices, garlic, and onion, and process the mixture until it is smooth.

   3. Add the chicken stock to the vegetable purée, and continue to process the mixture. The soup should be quite thick.

   4. Chill the soup thoroughly. Serve it cold with a dollop of yogurt and a sprinkling of green onions.

GAZPACHO

This is a very simple recipe. The secret is to chop each vegetable separately and roughly. If the soup is too thick when you are ready to serve it, dilute it with tomato juice.

1 small onion, peeled
2 small cucumbers, peeled and seeded
2 peppers (use a combination of colors—green,
    red, yellow)
6 tomatoes, seeded
5 cloves garlic, peeled
½ cup olive oil
1 hot pepper (chili or jalapeño) *or* Tabasco to
    taste
Freshly squeezed lemon juice (approximately the
    juice of ½ lemon)

1. Coarsely chop the onion in a food processor, and transfer the onion to a large bowl. Coarsely chop the cucumbers in the processor, and put them in the bowl with the chopped onion. Coarsely chop the peppers in the processor, and put them in the bowl with the other vegetables.

2. Chop 5 of the tomatoes, and put them in the bowl.

3. Put the garlic, 1 tomato, the olive oil, and the hot pepper or Tabasco in the processor, and process the ingredients until they are smooth. Add this mixture to the reserved chopped vegetables in the bowl, combining the ingredients well.

4. Taste the soup, and add lemon juice to taste.

5. Chill the soup for at least 3 hours.

GARLIC SOUP (AÏGO BOUÏDO) ⚞

The first time we were served this soup on the Costa del Sol, we couldn't figure out the ingredients. The garlic, due to its long cooking time, is very mellow.

1 head garlic (about 15 cloves), separated into
    cloves and bruised to open the skins
¼ teaspoon sage
¼ teaspoon thyme
½ bay leaf
2 whole cloves
Several sprigs parsley
3 tablespoons olive oil
2 quarts water
Salt to taste
Freshly ground pepper to taste
3 egg yolks
Toasted bread
Freshly grated hard cheese

1. In a large saucepan, combine the garlic, sage, thyme, bay leaf, cloves, parsley, and olive oil with the water, and bring the ingredients to a boil.

2. Lower the temperature, and simmer the soup for 30 minutes. Add the salt and pepper, and correct the seasonings.

3. Just before serving the soup, beat the egg yolks in a small bowl. Slowly add a little of the hot soup to the egg yolks, and continue beating the mixture until the ingredients are thoroughly blended. Then pour the remaining soup through a strainer into another saucepan, pressing hard on the garlic cloves. Add the warmed egg mixture to the strained soup.

4. Serve the soup immediately, placing on each portion a slice of toasted bread sprinkled with grated cheese.

FISH SOUP WITH AÏOLI

The best fish soup contains a great variety of seafood. Traditional local soups all around the Mediterranean are simply the result of the day's catch. We, too, have to make do with the "local catch" at our neighborhood fish market. You don't have to have lobster to dress up a plain fish soup, but a few scallops and two or three squid will enhance both the flavor and the look of the soup. Aïoli, a garlic sauce traditionally served with fish soup, also goes well with most vegetables.

AÏOLI

1 thick slice stale bread
3 tablespoons white-wine vinegar
6 cloves garlic, peeled
1 egg yolk
1 cup olive oil
2 tablespoons fresh lemon juice

FISH STOCK

1 pound fish frames, heads, and trimmings (reserved
   from the fillets; see "Fish Soup," below)
1 onion, peeled and coarsely chopped
1 tablespoon fresh lemon juice
1 cup white wine
4–5 cups cold water (enough to cover the fish)
Dash salt

FISH SOUP

1 onion, peeled and diced
1 or 2 leeks, trimmed, rinsed thoroughly, and
   cut into 1-inch pieces
2 cloves garlic, peeled and minced
2 tablespoons olive oil

continued on next page

3 medium tomatoes, seeded and chopped, *or* 1
    14-ounce can tomatoes, drained
⅓ cup white wine
Herbs (thyme, dill, *or* tarragon) to taste
4 cups fish stock (see above and below for
    ingredients and recipe, respectively)
1 pound firm, lean fish fillets such as halibut,
    red snapper, or grouper, cut into pieces
    (reserve the heads and frames for fish stock)
½ cup bay or sea scallops, cut into pieces if
    they are large
2 squid, cleaned and cut into pieces (see p. 138
    for the method)
Chopped parsley for garnish

    1. To make the aïoli, soak the bread in the vinegar, and squeeze the bread dry. Put the bread and garlic in a food processor, and process the ingredients into a paste. Add the egg yolk, and process the ingredients again to combine them. With the machine running, slowly add the olive oil through the feed tube. (If you are serving the aïoli with the fish soup, add a few tablespoons of the soup liquid to the sauce.) Process the lemon juice into the aïoli until it has the consistency of mayonnaise (which, in fact, it is).

    2. To make the fish stock, place in a large, heavy saucepan all the fish-stock ingredients. Bring the stock to a boil, skim it, reduce the heat, and simmer the stock for 30 minutes, uncovered. Strain the stock. (You should have about 4 cups.)

    3. To make the fish soup, in a soup pot, cook the onion, leeks, and garlic in the olive oil for about 5 minutes. Add the tomatoes. Bring the mixture to a boil, and add the white wine and herbs. Lower the temperature, and simmer the ingredients for 10 minutes. Add the stock and bring the soup to a simmer.

    4. Carefully add the fish to the soup pot, and cook the soup for another 5 minutes. Then stir in the scallops and squid, and cook the soup 5 minutes more or until the seafood is done but not overcooked.

    5. Serve the soup immediately, sprinkled with the chopped parsley and accompanied by the aïoli.

Entrées

SPANISH OMELET (PIPÉRADE) ◢

There are many versions of pipérade. This one is simple and hearty.

1 clove garlic, peeled and minced
1 small onion, peeled and chopped
3 tablespoons olive oil
2 tomatoes, seeded and chopped
1 green pepper, cored, seeded, and diced
2 slices Canadian bacon *or* lean ham, cut into
    small strips
5 eggs

1. In a large frying pan, Sauté the garlic and onion in 2 tablespoon of the olive oil until the onion is transcluscent. Add the tomatoes and green pepper. Stir the mixture over medium heat until it thickens and the onion is cooked. Pour the sauce in a bowl, and put it aside. In the same frying pan, quickly stir-fry the bacon or ham. Add this to the reserved sauce.

2. Break the eggs into a bowl, and whisk them lightly. Heat the last tablespoon of olive oil in the pan, and pour in the beaten eggs. Over medium heat, let the bottom of the omelet set. Pour the reserved sauce on top of eggs, and combine the sauce gently with the top layer of the eggs. Cover the frying pan, and cook the omelet until the eggs are almost firm. Slide the omelet out of the pan and onto a serving platter, or serve the omelet directly from the frying pan.

SEAFOOD "SHELLS" ✄

The casseroles or "shells" can be prepared ahead of time, then briefly heated in the microwave or oven. Parsley can be chopped in the food processor and the Parmesan grated without washing the appliance between each use.

3 cloves garlic, peeled
1 tablespoon olive oil
2 green onions (scallions)
¼ cup white wine
8 medium shrimp, peeled and deveined
1 cup scallops, cut into pieces
2 sprigs parsley, chopped
2 tablespoons freshly grated Parmesan

1. Mince the garlic in a food processor. Heat the olive oil in a frying pan. Add the garlic. Chop the green onions (scallions) in the food processor, and add them to the frying pan. Stir the mixture for 1 minute over low heat, and add the wine, shrimp, and scallops. Cook the mixture until shrimp just turn pink, 2 or 3 minutes.

2. Remove the seafood to a bowl. Strain the sauce, and reduce it to ¼ cup. Place 2 shrimp and equal portions of scallops in four oven-proof shells or small casseroles, sprinkling each portion with some chopped parsley and grated Parmesan. Spoon 1 tablespoon of the reduced sauce over each shell or casserole. Cover the dishes, and refrigerate them until you are almost ready to serve.

3. Just before serving, preheat the oven to 400°. Placing the shells or casseroles on a cookie sheet, bake them for 10 minutes or until they are bubbly. Or microwave them at medium for 2 minutes, stand time 3 minutes.

CHICKEN SALAD IN PITA POCKETS ✠

Pita, even when stuffed with a salad and taken to the workplace, keeps well. The ingredients of this chicken salad can vary but should always include garlic and onions.

2 skinned, cooked chicken breasts, diced
½ red or yellow pimiento, diced
12 chopped olives (good-quality canned black
   olives packed in oil or from the
   delicatessen)
2 green onions (scallions), minced
1 clove garlic, peeled and minced
1 tablespoon capers
2 tablespoons chopped parsley
¼ cup homemade mayonnaise made with olive
   oil (see pp. 125–126)
¼ cup low-fat or no-fat yogurt
4 whole-wheat pitas

1. Combine all of the ingredients except for the pitas.
2. Warm the pitas in an oven. Cut them in half, and open the pockets. Fill each pocket with some of the chicken salad.

MONKFISH MEDALLIONS WITH SKORDALIA ✍

Monkfish is a small coastal shark similar to the dogfish found in the eastern Mediterranean. Fish such as hake may be substituted for monkfish. The skordalia recipe yields about 1 cup of sauce, which will keep for several days in the refrigerator and may be served with vegetables as well as fish. This sauce can also be made with 2 large cold boiled potatoes instead of the bread.

SKORDALIA

2 large slices bread
6 cloves garlic, peeled
2 egg yolks
1 tablespoon fresh lemon juice
½ cup olive oil
Large bunch parsley

MONKFISH MEDALLIONS

1 clove garlic, peeled and chopped
2 green onions (scallions)
3 tablespoons olive oil
3 tablespoons flour
1 pound monkfish fillets, cut into ½-inch medallions

1. To make the skordalia, soak the bread in some water, and squeeze the bread dry.
2. In a food processor, mince the garlic. Add the bread, egg yolks, and lemon juice, and process the mixture for about 10 seconds. With the machine still running, slowly add the olive oil until the sauce thickens. Add the parsley to the skordalia, and process the sauce until the parsley is chopped and well incorporated.
3. In a skillet, sauté the garlic and green onions (scallions) in 2 tablespoons of the olive oil until the vegetables are soft. Add 1 tablespoon of oil to the skillet to heat.
4. Lightly flour the fish medallions, and add them to the hot oil. Turn the fish once. The fish is done when it loses its opacity.
5. Serve the medallions with the skordalia.

CHICKEN AND BULGUR ✗

All the ingredients in this dish are typical of Mediterranean cooking, but the recipe is our own.

1 chicken, cut into 6 serving pieces (2 breasts,
    2 legs, 2 thighs; reserve the wings and
    back for another use)
2 cloves garlic, peeled and chopped
3 tablespoons olive oil
1 large *or* 2 small onions, peeled and sliced
4 large tomatoes, chopped and seeded, *or* 1
    28-ounce can tomatoes
Rosemary to taste, chopped
½ cup white wine *or* red wine
½ cup bulgur

1. Remove the skin from the pieces of chicken.
2. In a large frying pan, sauté the garlic in the olive oil, add the onions, and sauté the vegetables until they are golden. Push the garlic and onions to the side of the pan, and in the same oil lightly sauté the chicken pieces. Add the tomatoes and rosemary to the pan, simmering the ingredients for 15 minutes. Add the wine to the pan, and cook the chicken for a few minutes more.
3. Remove the chicken, add the bulgur to the remaining sauce in the pan, and stir the ingredients well.
4. Replace the chicken in the pan on top of the bulgur mixture, and cover the pan. Simmer the chicken and bulgur for 20 minutes, adding water or more wine, if necessary.

VEAL SCALLOPINE AND PASTA WITH
WINE-AND-MUSHROOM SAUCE ⚡

*This dish can be prepared quickly and can serve either as a
simple, healthy meal at the end of a workday or as an elegant
dinner-party entrée. The sauce is used to flavor the pasta, which
should be cooked so that it is done at the same time the veal has
finished cooking.*

1 tablespoon butter
2 tablespoons olive oil
1 clove garlic, peeled and quartered
4 large mushrooms, sliced
10 fresh basil leaves, chopped, reserving some
    for garnish (if fresh basil is not available,
    substitute ¼ cup of chopped fresh
    parsley and 1 teaspoon of dried basil)
¾ cup white wine *or* vermouth
½ cup flour
1½ pounds veal scallopine
1 pound (16 ounces) linguine, cooked,
    drained, and tossed with 1 tablespoon
    olive oil
¼ cup freshly grated Parmesan

1. In a large frying pan, heat the butter and 1 tablespoon of the
olive oil. Add the garlic to the pan, and sauté the garlic for a few
minutes.

2. Add the mushrooms, and cook the vegetables for 2 minutes
more. Sprinkle half the basil over the ingredients.

3. Add ½ cup of the wine, and continue to cook the mixture until
the mushrooms are done, about 5 minutes. Remove the mixture to
a saucepan.

4. Add the remaining tablespoon of olive oil to the frying pan, and
turn the heat up to medium-high. Lightly flour the veal, add it to
the frying pan, and sauté the veal for 1 minute. Turn the veal over,
and sauté the meat on the other side for 1 minute more. Do not
overcook the veal.

5. Pour the mushroom-onion mixture over the meat, dribble another ¼ cup of wine over the ingredients, and cook the veal for 3 minutes more.

6. Remove the veal from the pan, and keep the meat warm. Add the linguine to the frying pan, mix the mushroom-onion sauce with the pasta, and arrange the pasta on a serving platter. Place the veal around the edge of the platter, and sprinkle the entire dish with the Parmesan and the reserved basil.

SEAFOOD PAELLA (PAELLA MARINERA) ⚖

When the rice dish paella spread from Valencia throughout Spain, cooks adapted it to include easy-to-obtain local ingredients. Some paellas contain sausage, lobster, and chicken. But we prefer the all-seafood paella.

½ cup olive oil
½ pound squid, cleaned and cut into pieces
    (see p. 138 for the method)
½ pound firm white fish (like halibut), skinned,
    boned, and cut into 1-inch cubes
1 onion, peeled and chopped
1 clove garlic, peeled and minced
2 tomatoes, chopped and seeded
½ teaspoon paprika
Hot red pepper, seeded and chopped, to taste (optional)
1½ cups rice
3½ cups water *or* fish stock
6 small shrimp, peeled and deveined
10 mussels, scrubbed and debearded

1. Heat the olive oil in a large, deep skillet that has a cover (we use an electric frying pan with a dome cover). To it add the squid and fish cubes. Sauté the seafood, and, when these turn golden, add the onion, garlic, tomatoes, paprika, and hot red pepper, if you wish. Cook the mixture for a few more minutes.

2. Add the rice and the water or fish stock. Cook the mixture rapidly for a few minutes. Add the shrimp and mussels. Lower the heat, cover the pan, and simmer the paella for 20 minutes or until all the liquid is absorbed and the rice is tender. By this time, the mussels will have opened (discard any that don't).

3. Either serve the paella in the cooking pan, or arrange it on a large platter with the shrimp and mussels decoratively placed around the edge of the dish.

BEANS AND SAUSAGE CASSEROLE

In this recipe, we have successfully eliminated most of the pork fat without sacrificing flavor. Note how little meat is necessary to satisfy a large appetite when the meat is combined with protein-rich beans. This dish tastes just as good the second day.

½ pound pork sausages
3 cups dried white beans, soaked overnight,
   drained, and rinsed
Salt to taste
1 clove garlic, peeled and chopped
1 tablespoon olive oil
1 onion, peeled and finely chopped
2 tablespoons chopped parsley
1 tablespoon tomato paste
½ cup water

1. Prick the sausages all over, and place them in a large saucepan in cold water to cover. Bring the water to a boil, and simmer the sausages for 10 minutes. Drain and rinse the sausages, and return them to the pan.

2. Add the beans to the pan, cover the beans and the sausages with water, and bring the ingredients to a boil. Simmer the beans and sausages for 2 hours, or cook them in a pressure cooker or a microwave oven according to the manufacturer's instructions (either of the latter methods will reduce cooking time significantly). When the beans are tender, add salt to taste.

3. In a large frying pan, sauté the garlic in the olive oil, and add the onion and parsley. Dilute the tomato paste with the water, and add this to the onion mixture. Simmer the ingredients for 20 minutes.

4. Drain the beans and sausages, and add them to the onion mixture, cooking and occasionally stirring the ingredients for another 20 minutes.

EGGPLANT AND GROUND-VEAL CASSEROLE (MOUSSAKA) ⟋

It is not unusual to discover vegetables other than eggplant in this layered casserole. We have been served versions that have included sautéed zucchini, sliced roasted potatoes, even artichokes. Sometimes, minced leftover lamb is substituted for the ground veal. The recipe that follows is rather traditional, but inventive cooks can make good use of leftovers in this dish.

2 eggplants (about 1 pound each), unpeeled
Salt
½–¾ cup plus 2 tablespoons olive oil
2 cloves garlic, peeled and chopped
½ onion, peeled and chopped
1 pound ground veal (if you prefer, you
    may use ground turkey instead)
2 tomatoes, seeded and chopped
2 tablespoons chopped parsley
Dash cinnamon
Dash nutmeg
¼ cup red wine
2 tablespoons olive oil *or* margarine
2 tablespoons flour
1½ cups milk
Salt to taste
Pepper to taste
Dash nutmeg
⅔ cup grated hard cheese (reserve 2
    tablespoons to finish the dish)
2 eggs, beaten

1. Cut the eggplants in ¼-inch-thick slices, place them on paper towels, and sprinkle them with salt. After 30 minutes, dry the eggplants with more paper towels. Do not rinse the slices.

2. In a large frying pan heat ½ cup of olive oil over medium-high heat. Add the eggplant slices to the pan, browning them on both

sides. Add more olive oil as needed. Drain the slices on paper towels, and keep the eggplant slices warm.

3. In another pan, heat the 2 tablespoons of olive oil, add the garlic and onion, and sauté the vegetables for a few minutes. Add the veal (or turkey), tomatoes, parsley, cinnamon, nutmeg, and red wine, and cook the mixture slowly for 30 minutes.

4. To make a béchamel (white sauce), in a saucepan heat the olive oil or margarine over medium heat, add the flour, and stir the roux for 1 minute. Quickly add the milk, and continue to stir. Bring the sauce to a boil, reduce the heat, and simmer the béchamel for 2 minutes, stirring it constantly. Add salt and pepper to taste as well as the nutmeg. Mix 2 or 3 spoonfuls of the béchamel sauce into the meat mixture.

5. In a lightly oiled casserole dish (approximately 11 × 8 inches), alternate layers of eggplant slices with the meat sauce (the eggplant slices should make up the bottom and top layers), sprinkling each layer with some of the cheese before adding another layer. Add the eggs to the béchamel, and pour the sauce evenly over the moussaka. Sprinkle the top of the moussaka with the reserved 2 tablespoons of cheese. Bake the casserole in a 350° oven for 45 minutes or until the top of the moussaka is golden.

CHICKEN COOKED WITH 30 CLOVES OF GARLIC ⚶

In this recipe, of which there are many versions, the large amount of garlic, cooked slowly, is not as overwhelming as you might think. Rather, the flavor is subtle and delicious.

2 tablespoons olive oil
1 chicken, cut into 8 serving pieces
1 onion, peeled and coarsely chopped
4 celery stalks with leaves, chopped
2 carrots, coarsely chopped
2 tablespoons parsley
30 cloves garlic (approximately 2 heads),
    unpeeled and slightly crushed
½ cup white wine *or* vermouth
1 teaspoon dried tarragon *or* thyme

   1. Pour the olive oil into a large frying pan, and heat the oil over medium-high heat. Add the chicken pieces to the hot oil, and lightly sauté the chicken.
   2. Place the onion, celery, carrots, and parsley in the bottom of a large casserole that has a tight-fitting lid. Put the sautéed chicken on top of the vegetables, surrounding the chicken with the garlic. Pour the wine or vermouth over the chicken, and sprinkle the chicken with the tarragon or thyme.
   3. Cover the casserole, and bake it in a moderate oven (325°) for 1½ hours without lifting the cover.
   4. Remove the casserole from the oven, uncover the dish, strain the juices (there will be a lot), and reduce the juices to a saucelike consistency. Place the sauce in a small serving bowl.
   5. Serve the chicken with the unskinned garlic cloves (the skins on the cloves of garlic are easily removed by the diner, and the garlic can be eaten as is with the chicken or spread on a piece of bread), and pass the sauce.

STUFFED SQUID ⚔

We find squid to be bland and, therefore, serve it cooked in a sauce or with an accompaniment. For plain fried squid, try a yogurt-garlic sauce. Although the following dish is more involved than fried squid, it is also tastier.

4 large squid or 8 small squid, cleaned (see p.
   138 for the method)
1 tablespoon plus ½ cup olive oil
1 tablespoon chopped parsley
2 cloves garlic, peeled and minced, plus 3
   cloves garlic, peeled
1 egg
¼ cup dry bread crumbs
⅓ cup grated hard cheese
Salt to taste
Freshly ground pepper to taste
1 tomato, seeded and chopped
¼ cup white wine

1. Chop the tentacles of the squid, leaving the rest of the squid whole. Mix the chopped squid with the 1 tablespoon of olive oil, the parsley, 1 peeled and minced garlic clove, and the egg. Add the bread crumbs and cheese. Season the stuffing with salt and pepper.

2. Lightly stuff the squid with the stuffing, and sew up the openings in the squid.

3. In a large frying pan, heat the ½ cup of olive oil, and, over medium heat, sauté the 3 peeled cloves of garlic. Discard the garlic after a few minutes. Brown the squid evenly, then add the tomato and the remaining clove of minced garlic. Cook the ingredients for a few minutes, add the wine to the frying pan, cover the pan, and simmer the squid for 30 minutes.

4. Just before you are ready to serve, remove the thread from the squid. Serve the squid either whole or sliced and arranged on a platter with the sauce.

SWORDFISH KEBABS

The firm flesh of the swordfish is ideal for kebabs. Do not overmarinate the fish; 1 hour is sufficient.

1½ pounds swordfish steaks, cut into large cubes
¼ cup olive oil
1 tablespoon fresh lemon juice
½ green pepper, seeded and cut into 1-inch
    squares
½ red pepper, seeded and cut into 1-inch
    squares
½ yellow pepper, seeded and cut into 1-inch
    squares
2 zucchini, thickly sliced, blanched in boiling
    water for 30 seconds, drained, and rinsed
    in cold water
2 tomatoes, cut into thick wedges
8 slices lemon
1 large onion, peeled and cut into wedges

1. Marinate the swordfish in the olive oil and lemon juice for 1 hour. Reserve the marinade.

2. Divide the fish, pepper squares, zucchini, tomatoes, lemon, and onion into 4 portions. Alternating the fish with the other ingredients, thread them on 4 sturdy skewers.

3. Brush the kebabs with the reserved marinade before placing them on the grill or in the broiler, basting them several times while they are cooking. Turn the kebabs once after 5 minutes. Cook the kebabs for another 5 to 10 minutes, depending on the temperature of the grill or broiler and on how close the kebabs are to the source of heat.

MACARONI AND CHOPPED-VEAL CASSEROLE (PASTITSIO) ⚄

Variations of this Greek staple are found in most Mediterranean countries. The casserole is easy to prepare, and the recipe can easily be doubled, tripled, or quadrupled. Because of the eggs, this dish does not freeze well, but it can be baked ahead of time and reheated in the oven (or in the microwave) just before serving it.

1 pound macaroni, preferably the long tube
   variety
2 tablespoons olive oil
1 pound ground veal *or* lean beef *or* turkey
Dash nutmeg
Dash cinnamon
1 onion, peeled and minced
2 tomatoes, seeded and chopped
2 tablespoons olive oil *or* margarine
2 tablespoons flour
1½ cups milk
Salt to taste
Pepper to taste
Dash nutmeg
2 eggs, beaten
⅔ cup grated hard cheese

1. Cook the macaroni according to the manufacturer's instructions, drain the pasta, and toss the pasta with 1 tablespoon of the olive oil.
2. Season the veal or beef or turkey with the nutmeg and cinnamon. Brown it in a large frying pan, and discard any rendered fat. In another pan, sauté the onion in 1 tablespoon of olive oil. Add the onion to the meat, then add the tomatoes. Simmer the ingredients for 20 minutes.
3. To make a béchamel (white sauce), in a saucepan heat the 2 tablespoons of olive oil or margarine over medium heat, add the flour, and stir the roux for 1 minute. Quickly add the milk, and continue to stir. Bring the sauce to a boil, reduce the heat, and simmer the

béchamel for 2 minutes, stirring it constantly. Add salt and pepper to taste as well as the nutmeg. Add 2 tablespoons of the béchamel to the meat mixture.

4. Oil a casserole dish. Put half the macaroni on the bottom of the casserole, and the meat sauce on top of the macaroni. Sprinkle the meat sauce with half of the cheese. Put the remaining macaroni over the cheese. Thoroughly combine the white sauce with the eggs, and pour the mixture over the top layer of macaroni. Sprinkle this last layer with the remaining half of the cheese.

5. Bake the casserole in a 350° oven for about 30 minutes or until the top of the casserole is browned.

STUFFED CABBAGE LEAVES ⚶

We always use the pressure cooker for this recipe, but it can just as easily be cooked on top of the stove or in the oven.

16 large cabbage leaves
1 onion, peeled and chopped
1 clove garlic, peeled and chopped
½ pound ground veal
¼ cup raw rice
3–4 fresh mint leaves
1 tablespoon chopped parsley
1 teaspoon chopped dill
Pinch cinnamon
1 tablespoon olive oil
2 tomatoes, seeded and chopped
1 cup tomato juice

1. Blanche the cabbage leaves in boiling water just enough to make them pliable. Drain them, and rinse them in cold water. Set them aside. Remove their tough stems.

2. Combine the onion and garlic.

3. Mix the veal with the rice, and add the onion and garlic.

4. Process the mint leaves, parsley, and dill in a food processor, and combine this with the meat mixture. Add the cinnamon and olive oil.

5. Using your hands, mix the ingredients well. Take the two largest cabbage leaves, and place them on the rack of your pressure cooker or on the bottom of a large pot. Divide the meat mixture into 14 equal portions, place a portion of meat on each of the remaining cabbage leaves, roll up each leaf egg-roll style, and hold the roll together with toothpicks.

6. Arrange the stuffed cabbage leaves in layers in the pressure cooker or pot. Add the tomatoes and tomato juice.

7. Pressure-cook the stuffed cabbage for 10 minutes, and allow pressure to drop naturally. Or cook the cabbage on top of the stove or in a 325° oven for about 1 to 1½ hours. If a lot of juice has accumulated at the bottom of the pot, remove the stuffed cabbage leaves to a serving platter, reduce the juices, and serve this sauce on the side.

SALMON STEAKS WITH ROTINI AND JULIENNED VEGETABLES ⚓

This dish has everything—color, shape, texture, aroma. The fish steaks can be poached in the microwave with excellent results. The vegetables can also be steamed in the microwave, then finished on top of the stove using a little of the fish poaching liquid to enhance their flavor.

1 pound rotini (corkscrew-shaped pasta)
3 tablespoons olive oil
2 small zucchini, sliced ¼-inch thick
2 carrots, peeled and julienned (cut into 2-inch matchstick strips)
½ head cauliflower, center portion, broken into small flowerets
1 stalk broccoli, broken into small flowerets
1 bunch dill
1 clove garlic, peeled and chopped
3 green onions (scallions)
½ cup white wine
4 salmon steaks, ¾-inch thick (about 6 ounces each)
1 teaspoon capers

1. Cook the rotini according to the manufacturer's directions. When the pasta is done, toss it with 1 tablespoon of the olive oil, and keep it warm.

2. Steam the zucchini, carrots, cauliflower, and broccoli separately, adding a few sprigs of dill to each vegetable during the steaming process and discarding them once the vegetables have been cooked.

3. While the pasta is cooking, pour the remaining 2 tablespoons of olive oil into a large glass baking dish. Add the garlic and ½-inch pieces of the white part of the green onions (scallions), chopping and reserving the green parts. Microwave the ingredients for 2 minutes at high. Add the wine and salmon steaks. Spoon the liquid over the fish. Place 1 sprig of dill (discarding the tough stem) on each steak.

Sprinkle the capers over the fish. Cover the dish, and microwave the fish for 5 minutes on high, stand time 3 minutes.

Or, to cook by conventional method, preheat oven to 325°. Sauté the garlic and onions in the olive oil in a saucepan until the vegetables are transluscent. Pour the ingredients into a glass baking dish, and prepare the fish as explained in the paragraph above. Cover the dish either with a fitted lid or with aluminum foil, and poach the fish in the oven for 15 minutes. Test for doneness by carefully flaking the inner portion of one of the pieces of fish. If it separates easily, it is done. Do not overcook the fish.

4. Pour the poaching liquid into a large skillet. Transfer all the vegetables to the reserved poaching liquid, and, on top of the stove, over high heat, reduce the liquid to a scant ½ cup.

5. Place the salmon on a large platter. With a slotted spoon, remove the vegetables from the poaching liquid, and arrange them attractively around the steaks.

6. Toss the rotini with the reserved reduced poaching liquid, and serve the pasta separately. To add color to the rotini, scatter the reserved chopped scallion greens over the pasta.

SALADE NIÇOISE ⚖

The success of this salad depends on the freshness of the vegetables. Good-quality tuna is also important.

1 7-ounce can white-tuna chunks packed in oil
1 small tin anchovies, drained, reserving 1
    tablespoon of the oil and 4 anchovies
1 tablespoon olive oil
2 tablespoons white-wine *or* red-wine vinegar
Salt to taste
Freshly ground pepper to taste
2 medium-sized boiled cold new potatoes,
    peeled and sliced
2 hard-boiled eggs, peeled and quartered
4 cups salad greens (romaine, red lettuce,
    Bibb, *and/or* spinach, in any combination)
½ pound green beans, trimmed and blanched
2 tomatoes, quartered and seeded
½ pound good-quality pitted black olives
2–3 tablespoons chopped fresh herbs
1 teaspoon capers

1. Drain the tuna, reserving the oil. Add the reserved oil from the tin of anchovies to the tuna oil. To the oils add the olive oil, wine vinegar, and salt and pepper to taste. In a medium bowl, flake the tuna into smaller pieces (but not very small), and set it aside.

2. Marinate the potatoes in the oil-vinegar dressing while preparing the other ingredients.

3. Cut the reserved anchovies in half, placing an anchovy on each egg quarter.

4. With a slotted spoon, remove the potatoes from the oil-vinegar dressing. Toss the salad greens with half of the dressing. Arrange the potatoes, tuna, eggs, anchovies, green beans, tomatoes, and olives on top of the greens, and pour the rest of the dressing over the salad. Sprinkle the dish with the fresh herbs and capers.

Grains and Pasta

WARM VEGETABLE-FETTUCCINE MOLD ⟋⟍

*Our vegetarian guests ask for seconds and thirds of this
rich-tasting dish. Since it is best served warm, not hot, the mold
can be made in advance and is thus perfect for a buffet, where it
will serve 12.*

30 spears fresh asparagus *or* 2 packages frozen asparagus
10 fresh snow peas *or* ½ package frozen snow
   peas, each pod cut in thirds
½ cup frozen peas
½ sweet red pepper, cored, seeded, and diced
2 cups broccoli flowerets
½ cup chicken stock
3 cloves garlic, peeled and minced
Red-pepper flakes to taste
½ cup low-fat or no-fat yogurt
5 eggs
¾ cup grated hard cheese
2 tablespoons chopped parsley
1–3 tablespoons olive oil
8 ounces fettuccine

   1. Cook the asparagus, snow peas, peas, sweet red pepper, and
broccoli flowerets separately until the vegetables are just *al dente.* Set
the vegetables aside.
   2. Thoroughly combine the chicken stock, garlic, red-pepper
flakes, and yogurt in a medium saucepan. Heat the ingredients over
medium-low heat, but do not boil them.
   3. In a bowl, combine the eggs, cheese, and parsley. Add the
heated stock mixture to these ingredients, and mix them well.
   4. In a medium frying pan, sauté the snow peas and sweet red
pepper in 1 to 2 tablespoons of the olive oil for 1 minute.
   5. In a large pot, cook the fettuccine, following the manufacturer's

instructions, until the pasta is *al dente*. Drain the fettucine, and put it in a large bowl. Mix the pasta with 1 tablespoon of the olive oil. Add the stock mixture, and fold in the peas, snow peas, and sweet red pepper.

6. Oil a round of wax paper that has the same diameter as the soufflé dish you will be using. (The dish should be approximately 8 to 9 inches in diameter and 4 inches deep.) Oil the soufflé dish. Place the wax paper in the bottom of the soufflé dish. Arrange the broccoli so that their tops are on the bottom of the dish. Place the asparagus tips down around the edge of the dish. Pour the fettuccine mixture into the center of the soufflé.

7. Place the dish in a larger pan, and fill this pan with 1 inch of boiling water. Put the fettuccine in a 350° oven for 45 minutes, adding boiling water, if necessary, to keep the water level 1 inch high. Then remove the pan with the water from the oven, returning the soufflé dish to the oven for 30 minutes more.

8. Remove the fettucine from the oven, and let it rest for 15 minutes before unmolding it. Run a knife around the edge of the soufflé dish, turn the dish upside down on a platter, and tap the dish all around until its contents unmold on the platter. Remove the wax paper from the top of the vegetable fettuccine and serve the dish warm.

COLD TRICOLORED PASTA SALAD ⚓

Other vegetables that could be added to this pasta salad are artichokes, broccoli, and peas. The salad will keep in the refrigerator for several days.

8 ounces tricolored pasta (wheels, shells, or
    rigatoni)
1 tablespoon plus ¼ cup olive oil
½ pound carrots, scrubbed and julienned (cut
    into 2-inch matchstick strips)
2 onions, peeled and cut into small wedges
¼ cup water

¼ cup white wine
Herbs (coriander seeds, fennel seeds, fresh or
   dried thyme, bay leaf) to taste
½ lemon, juiced
Chopped parsley

1. In a large pot, cook the pasta, following the manufacturer's instructions, until the pasta is *al dente*. Drain the pasta, put it in a large bowl, and mix it with the 1 tablespoon of olive oil.

2. Place in a medium saucepan the carrots, onions, water, wine, the ¼ cup of olive oil, and herbs, and cook these ingredients over medium heat for 5 minutes. The vegetables should not be soft.

3. Let the sauce cool, and then add the lemon juice. Combine the sauce with the pasta, sprinkle the dish with the parsley, and serve the salad cold.

TABBOULI

This hearty bulgur salad usually evokes cries of "What is this?" Not only is it good for you, but we can almost guarantee that everyone will like it.

1 cup bulgur
2 cups cold water
2 large, ripe tomatoes, seeded and chopped
2 cloves garlic, peeled and minced
1 large onion, peeled and finely chopped
1 large bunch parsley, finely chopped
6–8 fresh mint leaves, finely chopped
½ cup olive oil
⅓ cup fresh lemon juice

1. Soak the bulgur in the water for 1 hour. Drain the bulgur, and put it in a bowl.

2. Mix the tomatoes, garlic, onion, parsley, and mint with the bulgur.

3. In a small bowl, whisk together the olive oil and lemon juice. Just before serving, pour the olive-oil mixture over the bulgur mixture, and mix the ingredients thoroughly.

OATMEAL AND PLUMPED DRIED FRUIT

This dish provides a quick, hearty breakfast.

½ cup mixed dried fruit such as whole prunes,
    apricots, and peaches
1⅓ cups quick-cooking oatmeal (not instant)
3 cups hot water
Pinch cinnamon
Skim milk

1. In a 2-quart glass bowl, combine the dried fruit and the oatmeal. Pour the hot water over the oatmeal mixture, mix the ingredients thoroughly, and heat the cereal in the microwave at high for 4 to 5 minutes, watching the cereal carefully so that it doesn't boil over. (A piece of wax paper on top of the cereal keeps it from spattering.)

Or, to cook this dish on top of the stove, place the fruit in a saucepan, cover the fruit with the hot water, bring the liquid to a boil, remove the pan from the heat, and let it stand for 5 minutes. Add the oatmeal, and, over medium-low heat, bring the mixture to a simmer. Cook the oatmeal, uncovered, stirring it frequently, for 15 minutes. Let the oatmeal stand for 2 minutes. Stir it.

2. Serve the oatmeal with the cinnamon and some skim milk.

Vegetables and Salads

WHITE BEAN AND ONION SALAD ⟋⟍

This dish makes a good summer luncheon meal or a refreshing addition to a buffet. Fresh beans that have been soaked and cooked can be used instead of the canned beans.

1 28-ounce can white beans (Great Northern
    beans)
4 tablespoons olive oil
4 tablespoons fresh lemon juice
1 tablespoon red-wine vinegar
Salt to taste
Freshly ground pepper to taste
¼ cup chopped parsley
¼ cup chopped dill
¼ cup chopped mint leaves
1 large onion, peeled and thinly sliced
1 ripe but firm tomato, sliced
1 green pepper, cored, seeded, and sliced
Black olives for garnish
Lemon wedges for garnish

1. Rinse the beans, and drain them.
2. In a large bowl, whisk together the olive oil, lemon juice, vinegar, salt, and ground pepper. Add the beans to the bowl, and mix the ingredients well.
3. Add the parsley, dill, mint leaves, onion, tomato, and green pepper to the beans. Toss the salad.
4. Before serving the salad, garnish it with the olives and lemon wedges.

TURKISH-STYLE BEET SALAD ✗

In Turkey, this salad almost always appears as one of many small dishes served before the main course. Bread is used to soak up some of the salad marinade.

4–5 medium beets, trimmed and scrubbed
2 tablespoons olive oil
1 tablespoon mild wine vinegar
2 tablespoons fresh lemon juice
1 clove garlic, peeled and chopped
2 green onions (scallions), thinly sliced

1. In a saucepan, cook the beets in water to cover until they are tender (about 1 hour). With a slotted spoon, remove the beets from the pan to a bowl. Reduce the remaining liquid in the pan to ⅓ cup, strain the liquid, and reserve it. When the beets are cool enough to handle, slip off their skins, and thinly slice the beets.

2. To the reserved beet juice add the olive oil, vinegar, lemon juice, and garlic. Mix the ingredients well, and pour this sauce over the beets.

3. Refrigerate the beets until they are cold. Serve the chilled beets garnished with the sliced green onions.

RATATOUILLE ✗

There are many recipes for this traditional dish. Make it in large batches since it keeps well in the refrigerator and is good both hot or cold.

2 eggplants, about 1 pound each, sliced into
¼-inch rounds
Salt
2 cloves garlic, peeled and chopped
2 onions, peeled and sliced
1 cup olive oil (approximately)

6 medium zucchini, sliced into ½-inch rounds
1 pound tomatoes, chopped, *or* 1 20-ounce can
   tomatoes
2 green peppers, cored, seeded, and cut into
   1-inch pieces
Herbs of your choice to taste (rosemary, thyme,
   basil, *or* oregano)
½ lemon

1. Place the sliced eggplants on paper towels, sprinkle the slices with salt, and let them drain for 30 minutes. Pat them dry with more paper towels, and cut them into cubes. Set the cubes aside.

2. In a large frying pan, sauté the garlic and onions in ¼ cup of the olive oil until the vegetables are golden.

3. Add the zucchini, and continue cooking the mixture until the zucchini begin to soften.

4. In a separate frying pan, sauté the reserved eggplant cubes in ½ cup of the olive oil, adding more oil as needed, until the cubes begin to soften.

5. Gently mix the eggplant cubes and zucchini together in a large Dutch oven or kettle. Add the tomatoes, green peppers, and herbs.

6. Bring the vegetables to a boil, and stir the stew gently. Reduce the heat to a simmer, cover the pot, and cook the vegetables for 15 to 20 minutes or until they are done but not too soft. Uncover the pot, and stir the vegetables again, being careful not to mash them.

7. Raise the heat under the pot, and boil down the juices until they have almost evaporated. Squeeze the lemon over the ratatouille and serve the dish hot, or refrigerate the stew and serve it instead of a salad.

IMAM BAYILDI ✗

Imam Bayildi ("the priest fainted") refers to the tale of a Turkish religious leader (an imam*) who liked this dish so much that he fainted* (bayildi) *from pleasure upon tasting it. It is delicious and looks beautiful. Use small eggplants so that one-half is a single serving.*

4 long, small eggplants
Salt
1 large onion, peeled and thinly sliced
¼ cup olive oil
2 small tomatoes, seeded and chopped
½ cup chopped parsley
Pinch sugar
2 cloves garlic, peeled and minced
Salt to taste
2 tablespoons fresh lemon juice
1½ cups water

1. Peel the eggplants lengthwise in ½-inch strips. Cut each eggplant in half lengthwise. Make slits on the inner side of each eggplant half. Sprinkle the eggplant halves with salt, and let them stand 30 minutes. Mop up the accumulated moisture with paper towels.

2. In a large frying pan, sauté the onion in the olive oil for 5 minutes. Remove the onion to a bowl, and add to it the tomatoes, parsley, sugar, garlic, salt, and lemon juice.

3. Sauté the eggplants in the oil remaining in the frying pan. Arrange the 8 halves cut side up in the pan. Stuff the onion-tomato mixture into the slits in the eggplants, spreading the remaining mixture on top of them. Add the water to the pan, cover the pan, and cook the eggplants for about 45 minutes or until the eggplants are tender. If necessary, add more water to the pan during the cooking.

4. Remove the pan from the heat, and let the eggplants cool. Carefully remove the eggplants to a large platter, and serve the dish at room temperature.

EGGPLANT SALAD ⟋

This eggplant salad can also be used as a spread for crackers or bread.

3 eggplants, about 1 pound each
⅓ cup fresh lemon juice
⅓ cup olive oil
1 tablespoon red-wine vinegar
Pinch salt
Tomato wedges for garnish
Black olives for garnish
Chopped parsley for garnish

1. Score the eggplants in several places. Place them in a 350° oven for about 30 minutes or until their skin wrinkles. Cool the eggplants, and peel them. Then cut them in half, and remove as many seeds as possible. Discard the seeds, and coarsely chop the remaining eggplant pulp.

2. Place the eggplant pulp in a food processor or blender, and add the lemon juice, olive oil, vinegar, and salt. Process the ingredients until they are smooth.

3. Place the salad in a shallow bowl, garnishing the dish with the tomato wedges, black olives, and parsley.

BEET GREENS ✍

Most cooks discard the beet greens and only cook the beets, but the greens are simple to prepare and nutritious. In the Mediterranean region, beet greens as well as other greens gathered from the wild are cooked in the following manner.

Leaves and stems of 5–6 young beets
⅓ cup olive oil
⅓ lemon, juiced
1 clove garlic, peeled and crushed
1 cup water

1. Cut the beets from the stems, leaving 2 inches of stem attached to the beets. Reserve the beets for another use. Wash the leaves and stems several times in cold water, cut the stems into 1-inch pieces, and place them in the bottom of a large saucepan. Coarsely chop the leaves, and place them on top of the stems.

2. Add the olive oil, lemon juice, garlic, and water to the pan. Bring the ingredients to a boil, lower the heat to medium, cover the pan, and cook the greens for 20 minutes. Uncover the pan, and reduce the liquid to ½ cup.

3. Serve the greens warm or at room temperature.

Desserts

"OIL" CAKE ⚘

Our neighbor in Lindos, Greece, makes this cake and always gives us a large piece. We were surprised to find that she makes it with olive oil—a light-tasting one. This cake keeps very well.

1 cup light-tasting olive oil
1½ cups granulated sugar
1 tablespoon baking soda
2¼ cups plus 3 tablespoons flour
Dash cinnamon
Dash salt
1 orange *or* 1 lemon, juiced and the peel grated
1 tangerine, juiced and the peel grated
¾ cup raisins *or* currants
1 tablespoon brandy *or* other spirits

1. Preheat the oven to 350°.
2. In a large bowl, beat together the oil and the sugar. In another bowl, sift together the baking soda, 2¼ cups of flour, the cinnamon, and salt.
3. To the oil-sugar mixture, add the sifted ingredients alternately with the orange-tangerine juice or the lemon-tangerine juice.
4. Coat the raisins or currants with the 3 tablespoons flour, and add them to the batter along with the grated orange or lemon peel and the grated tangerine peel. Stir in the brandy or other spirits.
5. Pour the batter into an oiled 8 × 8-inch square baking pan, put the pan in the oven, and bake the cake for about 1 hour or until a wooden toothpick inserted into the cake comes out clean.

SEMOLINA PUDDING ✗

This pudding is satisfyingly filling at the end of a light meal. For children, substitute vanilla or another flavoring for the rum.

⅓ cup raisins
Warm water
2 tablespoons flour
2 cups milk
Pinch salt
⅓ cup semolina
⅔ cup granulated sugar
1 tablespoon butter *or* scant 1 tablespoon oil
1 tablespoon rum
Grated peel of 1 orange
2 eggs, beaten
Cinnamon

1. Preheat the oven to 350°.
2. Soak the raisins in warm water to cover for 15 minutes. Drain them, dry them, coat them with the flour, and set them aside.
3. In a saucepan, bring the milk and salt almost to a boil, add the semolina, and stir the mixture rapidly and constantly with a wooden spoon until the semolina thickens and comes away from the sides of the pan.
4. Remove the saucepan from the heat, and add the sugar, butter or oil, and rum, stirring the mixture constantly. Add the orange peel and the reserved raisins, and combine the ingredients well.
5. Beat the eggs into the semolina, pour the pudding into an oiled 6-cup mold or into 6 oiled 1-cup molds, place the pudding in the oven, and bake it for 40 minutes.
6. Remove the pudding from the oven, and bring it to room temperature. Refrigerate the pudding. Serve the pudding unmolded or in individual molds sprinkled with cinnamon.

RASPBERRIES IN CHAMPAGNE ⁄⌐

This is an elegant, light dessert, easily assembled at the last minute.

1 pint raspberries, cleaned just before serving
1 cup chilled champagne
4 sprigs fresh mint

1. Divide the raspberries evenly among 4 long-stemmed glasses.
2. Pour ¼ cup of champagne into each glass over the raspberries.
3. Decorate each serving with a sprig of mint.

Short Bibliography

There are many excellent nutrition books that include menus and recipes for healthful food. The list that follows should be helpful to anyone interested in adopting a health-enhancing diet. We culled this list from over fifty titles currently available in bookstores and libraries. Included are books that specifically address the question of diet and cancer. Jane Brody, the *New York Times*'s Personal Health columnist, has produced a thoughtful and exhaustive study that answers many questions about balancing carbohydrates and proteins, and provides a wealth of healthful recipes. *The American Heart Association Cookbook* will be of special interest to people with high blood pressure and other heart diseases as well as to those concerned about the dietary prevention of cardiovascular diseases.

Alabaster, Oliver, M.D. *The Power of Prevention*. New York: Simon and Schuster, 1986.

The American Heart Association Cookbook, 4th ed. New York: David McKay, 1984.

Brody, Jane. *Jane Brody's Good Food Book*. New York: Norton, 1985.

Davidson, Alan. *Mediterranean Seafood*. Baltimore: Penguin, 1972.

Martin, Alice A., and Frances Tenenbaum. *Diet against Disease*. Boston: Houghton Mifflin, 1980.

Ornish, Dean, M.D. *Stress, Diet, and Your Heart*. New York: Holt, Rinehart & Winston, 1982.

White, Kristin. *Diet and Cancer*. New York: Bantam, 1984.

Wolfert, Paula. *Mediterranean Cooking*. New York: Ecco, 1985.

Notes

Introduction

1. World Health Organization, *World Health Statistics Annual* (Geneva, 1984). This is the most accurate comparative index of contemporary international health statistics.
2. World Health Organization Expert Committee on Cardiovascular Disease, *Prevention of Coronary Heart Disease,* WHO Technical Report Series, no. 678 (Geneva, 1982), p. 21.
3. Elizabet Helsing, "Malnutrition in an Affluent Society," *World Health* (October 1984): 14.
4. Christos Aravanis and Paul J. Ioannidis, "Nutritional Factors and Cardiovascular Diseases in the Greek Island Heart Study," in *Nutritional Prevention of Cardiovascular Disease*, ed. W. Lovenberg and Y. Yamori (New York: Academic Press, 1984).

Chapter 1

1. P. L. MacKendrick and V. M. Scramuzza, *The Ancient World* (New York: Holt, Rinehart & Winston, 1958), p. 175.
2. R. Carrington, *The Mediterranean: Cradle of Western Culture* (New York: Viking, 1971), p. 16.
3. MacKendrick and Scramuzza, pp. 4, 10, 16, 22, 175, 194–195, 464–465.

Chapter 2

1. Antonia Trichopoulou, "The Changing Pattern of Nutrition and Disease Incidence in Greece," paper presented at the Society of Nutrition and Research, Copenhagen, March 1985.
2. Italian Central Statistical Institute, "North-South Regional Variations of Gastro-Intestinal Cancer and Circulatory Disease," Vol. XXIII (Rome, 1978); compiled for the authors by Dr. James Hanley of the World Health Organization, Geneva.
3. World Health Organization, *World Health Statistics Annual* (Geneva, 1984), adjusted to January 1986, by WHO Statistics Division, Geneva.
4. *Ibid.*, p. 180.
5. *Ibid.*, pp. 184, 226, 250.
6. Italian Central Statistical Institute, *op. cit.*
7. Christos Aravanis and Paul J. Ioannidis, "Nutritional Factors and Cardiovascular Diseases in the Greek Island Heart Study," in *Nutritional Prevention of Cardiovascular Disease*, ed. W. Lovenberg and Y. Yamori (New York: Academic Press, 1984), pp. 125–135.
8. The Greek island study was undertaken within the framework of a larger international study: A. Keys *et al.*, *Seven Countries: A Multivariate Analysis of Death and Coronary Heart Disease* (Cambridge: Harvard University Press, 1980). The Greek researchers collected 224 daily food samples from Crete and 280 samples from Corfu at the beginning of the study, and 216 samples from Crete and 224 from Corfu at the end of the research. Detailed records of the dietary role of the foods were maintained on an annual basis. Mortality was followed annually and was based on the best possible information on the actual cause of death.
9. Statistical methodologies employed included frequency and significance controls derived from Student's t test and Cohran's t test. In addition, both constant and temporal intracohort differences were assessed for significance by the chi-square test. It should be noted that the coordinators of the parent seven-nation study required each separate research project to follow the most rigorous internationally recognized standards of statistical analysis so that the combined data could be rationally compared.
10. A. S. St. Leger, A. Z. Cochrane, and F. Moore, "Factors Associated with Cardiac Mortality in Developed Countries with Particular Reference to the Consumption of Wine," *Lancet* (May 12, 1979): 1017–1020. This was the first major international epidemiological survey to identify the apparent coronary health benefits of moderate wine consumption.
11. O. Manousos *et al.*, "Diet and Colorectal Cancer: A Case-Control Study in Greece," *International Journal of Cancer* 32 (1983): 1–5.
12. *Ibid.*, 3–5.
13. *Ibid.*, 5.
14. Italian Central Statistical Institute, *op. cit.*
15. Major similar studies include D. Trichopoulos *et al.*, "Diet and Cancer of the

Stomach: A Case-Control Study in Greece," *International Journal of Cancer* 36 (1985): 291–297, and T. Hirayama, "Epidemiology of Stomach Cancer in Japan with Special Reference to the Strategy for the Primary Prevention," *Japanese Journal of Clinical Oncology* 14, no. 2 (1984): 159–168.

16. Trichopoulou, *op. cit.*

17. *Ibid.*, 1, Table 1.

18. S. M. Grundy, "Comparison of Monounsaturated Fatty Acids and Carbohydrates for Lowering Plasma Cholesterol," *New England Journal of Medicine* 314, no. 12 (March 20, 1986): 745–748. In his introduction, Grundy states: "In countries such as Greece and in southern Italy, the traditional diet is high in olive oil, and total intake of fat can be high. In these countries, however, both the levels of plasma cholesterol and the rates of coronary heart disease are relatively low."

19. World Health Organization, pp. 216, 228.

20. Trichopoulou, p. 3.

21. *Ibid.* Trichopoulou states: "Furthermore, studies in [urban] children have shown that blood pressure and obesity indices are higher in Greece than in other European countries, predicting an ominous future if these trends continue and are not corrected with the appropriate preventative measures."

22. *Ibid.*, Fig. 4: "Age Adjusted Mortality (per 100,000) for Diabetes Mellitus in Greece by Gender, 1969–80"; and Fig. 5: "Standardized Mortality from Diabetes Mellitus in Urban, Semiurban, and Rural Areas of Greece by Gender, 1983." Based on these data, Trichopoulou states: "It can be seen, once again, how well the time and place differentials of diabetes mellitus mortality reflect the dietary patterns and their consequences on health and disease."

23. E. Velonakis *et al.*, "Epidemiological Characteristics of Diabetes Mellitus in Greece" (in Greek with English summary), *Ippokrates* 11 (1983): 257–264.

Chapter 3

1. S. M. Grundy *et al.*, "Rationale of the Diet-Heart Statement of the American Heart Association, Report of Nutrition Committee," *Circulation* 65, no. 4 (1982): 839–854.

2. W. B. Kannel and J. Gordon, eds., *Some Characteristics Related to the Incidence of Cardiovascular Disease and Death: Framingham Study, 16-Year Follow-up* (Washington, D.C.: U.S. Government Printing Office, 1970, 1974, 1979, 1983).

3. World Health Organization Expert Committee on Cardiovascular Disease, *Prevention of Coronary Heart Disease*, WHO Technical Report Series, no. 678 (Geneva, 1982), pp. 14–15.

4. Oliver Alabaster, *The Power of Prevention* (New York: Simon and Schuster, 1986), p. 73.

5. National Institutes of Health Consensus Development Conference, "Lowering

Blood Cholesterol to Prevent Heart Disease," *Journal of the American Medical Association* 253 (1985): 2080–2086, and J. Stamler, D. Wentworth, and J. D. Neaton, "Is the Relationship between Serum Cholesterol and Risk of Premature Death from Coronary Heart Disease Continuous and Graded?" *Journal of the American Medical Association* 256 (1986): 2823–2828.

6. Refined statistical estimate of the American Heart Association (AHA), National Center, Dallas, Texas. Announcing the AHA's most recent dietary guidelines in August 1986, the chairman of the association's National Nutritional Committee, Dr. John La Rosa, stated: "As many as 1.5 million Americans will have a heart attack this year, and about 550,000 of them will die. Improved nutrition remains one of the keys to improved health and fewer lives lost to cardiovascular disease and stroke."

7. Grundy *et al.*, 845A.

8. La Rosa, *op. cit.* In its 1985 Dietary Guidelines, the AHA recommends that total calories from fat should be reduced to "less than 30 percent."

9. Alabaster, pp. 38–39. With other international cancer experts, Alabaster recommends the following dietary changes: reduction of fat to 20 percent of daily calories; increased intake of dietary fiber; increased intake of beta-carotene-rich and cruciferous fruits and vegetables; increased intake of whole-grain cereals; maintenance of optimal weight; and avoidance of barbecued, smoked, and salt-cured foods. The 1986 Dietary Guidelines of the National Cancer Institute present similar recommendations.

10. B. Armstrong and R. Doll, "Environmental Factors and Cancer Incidence and Mortality in Different Countries, with Special Reference to Dietary Practices," *International Journal of Cancer* 15 (1975): 617–631; S. A. Tornberg *et al.*, "Risks of Cancer of the Colon and Rectum in Relation to Serum Cholesterol and Beta-Lipoproteins," *New England Journal of Medicine* 315, no. 26 (December 25, 1986): 1629–1633; and G. A. Mannes *et al.*, "Relation between the Frequency of Colorectal Adenoma and the Serum Cholesterol Level," *New England Journal of Medicine* 315, no. 26 (December 25, 1986): 1634–1638.

11. If you are interested in reviewing some of the fundamental studies on this subject, see N. D. Nigro *et al.*, *Journal of the National Cancer Institute* 54 (1975): 439–442; B. S. Reddy *et al.*, *Journal of the National Cancer Institute* 52 (1974): 507–511; and B. R. Bansal *et al.*, *Cancer Research* 38 (1978): 293–303.

12. Alabaster p. 84.

13. Interviewed by Margie Patlak in the *Washington Post* (April 18, 1986).

14. Antonia Trichopoulou, "The Changing Pattern of Nutrition and Disease Incidence in Greece," paper presented at the Society of Nutrition and Research, Copenhagen, March 1985.

15. Alabaster, pp. 87–88.

16. In this regard, the Public Health Service of the National Institutes of Health concurs. See U.S. Department of Health and Human Services, "Diet, Nutrition and Cancer Prevention: A Guide to Food Choices," NIH Publication no. 85-2711 (November 1984).

17. Kannel and Gordon, *op. cit.*

18. Taken from research conducted by the Center for Science in the Public Interest, as reported in the *Washington Post* (April 12, 1986): A23.

Chapter 4

1. Scott M. Grundy, "Comparison of Monounsaturated Fatty Acids and Carbohydrates for Lowering Plasma Cholesterol," *New England Journal of Medicine* 314, no. 12 (March 20, 1986): 745–748, and R. Levy *et al.*, eds., *Nutrition, Lipids, and Coronary Heart Disease* (New York: Raven Press, 1979), pp. 26–88.
2. World Health Organization Expert Committee on Cardiovascular Disease, *Prevention of Coronary Heart Disease*, WHO Technical Report Series, no. 678 (Geneva, 1982), p. 21.
3. J. Eaton and E. Graf, *Cancer* 56, no. 4 (1985): 717.
4. Paul A. Lachance, "Please Pass the Bread," *Professional Nutritionist* 14, no. 2 (Spring 1982): 7–10.
5. Jane Brody, *Jane Brody's Good Food Book: Living the High-Carbohydrate Way* (New York: Norton, 1985), pp. 18–26.
6. *Ibid*, p. 13.
7. Lachance, *op. cit.*
8. S. M. Grundy *et al.*, "Rationale of the Diet-Heart Statement of the American Heart Association, Report of the Nutrition Committee," *Circulation* 65, no. 4 (1982): 841A.
9. U.S. Department of Agriculture and U.S. Department of Health and Human Services, *Dietary Guidelines for Americans* (Washington, D.C., August 1985); P. Greenwald and E. Lanza, "Dietary Fiber and Colon Cancer," *Contemporary Nutrition* 11, no. 1 (1986); G. V. Vahouny and D. Kritchevsky, eds., *Dietary Fiber in Health and Disease* (New York: Plenum, 1982).
10. O. Manousos *et al.*, "Diet and Colorectal Cancer: A Case-Control Study in Greece," *International Journal of Cancer* 32 (1983): 3–5.
11. J. W. Anderson *et al.*, "Hypocholesterolemic Effects of Oat-Bran or Bean Intake for Hypercholesterolemic Men," *American Journal of Clinical Nutrition* 40 (1984): 1146–1155.
12. World Health Organization Expert Committee on Cardiovascular Disease, p. 21.

Chapter 5

1. Scott M. Grundy, "Comparison of Monounsaturated Fatty Acids and Carbohydrates for Lowering Plasma Cholesterol," *New England Journal of Medicine* 314, no. 12 (March 20, 1986): 745–748. Also see: R. P. Mensink and M. B. Katahn, "Effect of monounsaturated fatty acids vs. complex carbohydrates on

high-density lipoproteins in healthly men and women," *The Lancet,* January 17, 1987, pp. 122–124.

2. Grundy, as quoted in the *New York Times* (March 20, 1986): A14.

3. For an interesting discussion of the free-radical–polyunsaturated-fats interaction, see Oliver Alabaster, *What You Can Do to Prevent Cancer* (New York: Simon and Schuster, 1985), pp. 151–153. Also see Charles B. Simone, *Cancer and Nutrition* (New York: McGraw-Hill, 1983), pp. 44–52; L. Reich and S. S. Stivala, in *Autoxidation of Hydrocarbons and Polyoletins* (New York: Dekker, 1969); and W. O. Lundberg, in *Autoxidation and Antioxidants,* Vol. I (New York: Wiley, 1961).

4. Grundy, as quoted in the *Associated Press Medical News Features* (March 1986).

5. Grundy, "Comparison . . . ," 746–747.

6. Publio Viola and Mirella Audisio, "Olive Oil and Health," research compendium presented at the Third International Congress on the Biological Value of Olive Oil, Canea, Crete, Greece, September 1980 (updated for distribution April 1986). This compendium is the most inclusive summary of international research on the health benefits of olive oil. The study is available through the International Olive Oil Council, Bartucci-Samuel, Inc., 1 World Trade Center, Suite 7967, New York, NY 10048.

7. *Ibid.,* pp. 10–11. Also see F. C. Jager, "Linoleic Acid and Vitamin E," in *The Role of Fats in Human Nutrition,* ed. A. J. Vergroese (London: Academic Press, 1975), pp. 176–181.

Chapter 6

1. Giorgio Lolli *et al., Alcohol in Italian Culture* (Glencoe, Ill.: Free Press, 1958); Pablo S. Lucia, *Alcohol and Civilization* (New York: McGraw-Hill, 1963); R. O'Brien and M. Chafetz, *The Encyclopedia of Alcoholism* (New York: Facts on File, 1982), pp. 15–37.

2. P. L. MacKendrick and V. M. Scramuzza, *The Ancient World* (New York: Holt, Rinehart and Winston, 1958), pp. 148–156.

3. Winegrowers of California, *Wine and America* (Emeryville, Calif., 1986), p. 10.

4. A. S. St. Leger, A. Z. Cochrane, and F. Moore, "Factors Associated with Cardiac Mortality in Developed Countries with Particular Reference to the Consumption of Wine," *Lancet* (May 12, 1979): 1017–1020.

5. *Ibid.,* 1018.

6. W. C. Blackwelder *et al.,* "Alcohol and Mortality: The Honolulu Heart Study," *American Journal of Medicine* 68 (1980): 164–169.

7. R. E. La Porte *et al.,* "Alcohol, Coronary Heart Disease, and Total Mortality," *Recent Developments in Alcoholism* 3 (1986): 156–163. Also see R. E. La Porte

et al., "The Relationship of Alcohol Consumption to Atherosclerotic Heart Disease," *Preventive Medicine* 9 (1980): 22–40.

8. A. L. Klatsky *et al.*, "Alcohol and Mortality: A Ten-Year Kaiser-Permanente Experience," *Annals of Internal Medicine* 95 (1981): 139–145.

9. St. Leger, Cochrane, and Moore, 1017. St. Leger and his colleagues measured the correlation coefficients between death rates and the following variables: numbers of doctors and nurses; gross national product; population density; cigarette smoking; alcohol consumption, including wine, beer, and spirits; average daily calories in diet; total dietary fat, including total saturated, polyunsaturated, and monounsaturated dietary fat; and, finally, Key's Predictive Equation for serum cholesterol. According to the authors of the study: "The principal finding is a strong and specific negative association between ischemic heart-disease deaths and alcohol consumption. This is shown to be wholly attributable to wine consumption."

10. C. A. Camargo *et al.*, "The Effect of Moderate Alcohol Intake on Serum Apolipoproteins A-I and A-II," *Journal of the American Medical Association* 253, no. 19 (1985): 2854–2857.

11. A. Lasserre *et al.*, "Mortality Rates by Cirrhosis, Chronic Alcoholism, and by Esophagus Cancer in France, 1954–1963," in *Trends in Cancer Incidence*, ed. Knut Magnus (New York: Hemisphere, 1982), p. 69.

12. Winegrowers of California, p. 27.

13. Matheson & Matheson, Inc., *A Survey of Wine Service in Hospitals in the Top Metropolitan Areas of the United States* (San Francisco: Matheson & Matheson, September 1985).

14. R. Kastenbaum and B. L. Mishara, *Alcohol and Old Age* (Orlando, Fla.: Grune & Stratton, 1980).

15. Phyllis C. Richman, "Convening to Promote the Essence of the Mediterranean Diet," *Washington Post* (December 11, 1985): E1, E8.

Chapter 7

1. Charles B. Simone, *Cancer and Nutrition* (New York: McGraw-Hill, 1983), pp. 49, 63–65, and R. Peto *et al.*, "Can Dietary Beta-Carotene Materially Reduce Human Cancer Rates?" *Nature* 290, 201.

2. See Oliver Alabaster, *The Power of Prevention* (New York: Simon and Schuster, 1986), pp. 133–137. Alabaster presents a detailed summary of recent research on the protective properties of dietary beta-carotene, including the work of the following researchers: R. MacLennan *et al.*, *International Journal of Cancer* 20 (1977): 854–860; A. Gregor *et al.*, *Nutrition and Cancer* 2 (1980): 93–97; P. G. Smith and H. Jick, *Cancer* 42 (1978): 808–811; R. B. Shekelle *et al.*, *Lancet* 2 (1981): 1185–1189; E. L. Wynder and I. J. Bross, *Cancer* 14 (1961): 389–413;

C. Mettlin *et al.*, *Nutrition and Cancer* 2 (1981): 143–147; D. L. McCormick, F. J. Burns, and R. E. Albert, *Journal of the National Cancer Institute* 66 (1981): 559–564; M. M. Mathews-Roth, *Oncology* 39 (1982): 33–37.

3. Committee on Diet, Nutrition, and Cancer, Assembly of Life Sciences, Nutritional Research Council, National Academy of Sciences, *Diet, Nutrition, and Cancer* (Washington, D.C.: National Academy Press, 1982). The recommendations in this study have been summarized in the U.S. Department of Health and Human Services' "Diet, Nutrition and Cancer Prevention: A Guide to Food Choices," NIH Publication no. 85-2711 (November 1984).

4. World Health Organization, *World Health Statistics Annual* (Geneva, 1984), p. 227.

5. W. L. Wattenberg *et al.*, "Dietary Constituents Altering the Response to Chemical Carcinogens," *Proceedings of the Federation of American Societies of Experimental Biology* 32 (1976): 1862.

6. T. Colin Campbell, interviewed by Eric Levin in *People* (June 1985).

7. Alabaster, p. 198, and S. Graham *et al.*, *Cancer* 30 (1972): 927–938.

8. James Cerda, quoted by Sarah Fritschner in the *Washington Post* (January 9, 1983).

Chapter 8

1. Richard Carrington, *The Mediterranean: Cradle of Western Culture* (New York: Viking, 1971), pp. 50–51.

2. D. Kromhout *et al.*, "The Inverse Relation between Fish Consumption and 20-Year Mortality from Coronary Heart Disease," *New England Journal of Medicine* 312 (1985): 1205–1209. Also see American Heart Association, *Science Writers Forum*, Research Report no. 5 (January 25–28, 1982).

3. B. E. Phillipson *et al.*, "Reduction of Plasma Lipids, Lipoproteins, and Apoproteins by Dietary Fish Oils in Patients with Hypertriglyceridemia," *New England Journal of Medicine* 312 (1985): 1210–1216.

4. American Heart Association, *Science Writers Forum, Research Report no. 6* (December 1982), p. 5.

5. Phillipson *et al.*, *op. cit.*

6. Kromhout *et al.*, *op. cit.*; Phillipson *et al.*, *op. cit.*

7. Kromhout *et al.*, *op. cit.*

8. A. Trichopoulou, "The Changing Pattern of Nutrition and Disease Incidence in Greece," paper presented at the Society of Nutrition and Research, Copenhagen, March 1985.

Chapter 9

1. M. H. Brodnitz *et al.*, "Flavor Components of Garlic Extract," *Journal of Agricultural Food Chemistry* 19 (1971): 273–275. Also see Eric Block, "The Chemistry of Garlic and Onions," *Scientific American* (May 1983): 114–120.

2. *Tufts University Diet and Nutrition Letter* 3, no. 6 (August 1985): 7. Bordia's original findings appear in A. K. Bordia and S. K. Verma, "Garlic on the Reversibility of Experimental Atherosclerosis," *Indian Heart Journal* 30 (1978): 47, and A. K. Bordia *et al.*, "Effects of Essential Oils of Garlic and Onion on Alimentary Hyperlipemia," *Atherosclerosis* 21 (1975): 15–19.

3. R. C. Jain, "Effect of Garlic on Serum Lipids, Coagulability and Fibrinolytic Activity," *American Journal of Clinical Nutrition* 30 (1977): 1380.

4. Bordia and Verma, *op. cit.*

5. R. Bakish and M. I. D. Chughtai, "Influence of Garlic on Serum Cholesterol, Serum Triglycerides, Serum Total Lipids, and Serum Glucose in Human Subjects" (in English), *Die Nahrung* 28, no. 2 (1984): 159–163.

6. Dr. Myung Chi, quoted by Dorothy Foster Sly in the *Professional Nutritionist* (August 1983): 22.

7. *Ibid.*

8. B. H. S. Lau, M. A. Adetumbi, and A. Sanchez, "*Allium Satvium* (Garlic) and Atherosclerosis: A Review," *Nutrition Research* 3 (1983): 119.

9. G. S. Sainani, "Dietary Garlic, Onion and Some Coagulation Parameters in Jain Community," *Journal of the Association of Physicians of India* 27 (1979): 707.

10. James L. Catalfamo, quoted by Ann M. Williams in "Garlic Yields Anti-Clotting Compound," *American Heart Association, Cardiovascular Research Report* (Summer 1985): 7.

11. Isabella Lipinska, quoted in *Tufts University Diet and Nutrition Letter* 3, no. 6 (August 1985): 7.

12. *Science Digest* (April 1980): 20.

Chapter 10

1. Center for Science and the Public Interest, as reported by Colman McCarthy, "Really Greasy Spoons," *Washington Post* (April 12, 1986): op. ed. p.

2. American Heart Association Health News Center, Dallas, Texas.

3. World Health Organization, *World Health Statistics Annual* (Geneva, 1984), pp. 181, 229, 259.

4. C. D. Jenkins, "Recent Evidence Supporting Psychologic and Social Risk Factors for Coronary Disease," *New England Journal of Medicine* 294 (1976): 987–994, 1033–1038; R. S. Eliot, *Stress and the Major Cardiovascular Disorders* (Mount Kisco, N.Y.: Futura Publishing, 1979); and Dean Ornish, *Stress, Diet, and Your Heart* (New York: Holt, Rinehart & Winston, 1982).

5. Ornish, pp. 41–63.
6. J. I. Haft and K. Fani, "Intravascular Platelet Aggregation in the Heart Induced by Stress," *Circulation* 47 (1973): 353–358, and J. I. Haft and Y. S. Arkel, "Effect of Emotional Stress on Platelet Aggregation in the Heart," *Chest* 70 (1976): 501.
7. Ornish, pp. 49–155, and J. Stamler, "Lifestyles, Major Risk Factors, Proof and Public Policy," *Circulation* 58 (1978): 3–19.
8. Hans Selye, *Stress without Distress* (New York: Lippincott, 1978), and *id.*, *Selye's Guide to Stress Research*, Vol. 1 (New York: Van Nostrand Reinhold, 1980).

Chapter 11

1. World Health Organization, *World Health Statistics Annual* (Geneva, 1984). It is instructive to compare the cardiovascular health statistics of Italy, Greece, Spain, Israel, and Turkey with those of Great Britain, West Germany, the Benelux countries, and Scandinavia.
2. *Ibid.*, pp. 229, 253. Cardiovascular health has been connected to both diet and stress-management strategies by Selye, Ornish, and others. Given the demographics of the contemporary Mediterranean world, urban centers now account for over half the region's population, yet these cities have a relatively low rate of cardiovascular disease. But the socially isolated suburban sprawl typical of the United States is almost unknown in southern Europe.
3. K. Orth-Gomer and A. Ahlbom, "Impact of Psychological Stress on Ischemic Heart Disease When Controlling for Conventional Risk Indicators," *Journal of Human Stress* 6 (1980): 7–15.
4. R. S. Paffenbarger and W. E. Hale, "Work Activity and Coronary Heart Mortality," *New England Journal of Medicine* 292 (1975): 545, and R. S. Paffenbarger et al., "Physical Activity as an Index of Heart Attack Risk in College Alumni," *American Journal of Epidemiology* 108 (1978): 161–175.
5. For an excellent overview of the health benefits of exercise, see Dean Ornish, *Stress, Diet, and Your Heart* (New York: Holt, Rinehart & Winston, 1982), and G. S. Thomas, P. R. Lee, P. Franks, and R. S. Paffenbarger, *Exercise and Health: The Evidence and the Implications* (Cambridge, Mass.: Oelgeschlager, Gunn & Hain, 1981).
6. Lorelei DiSogra and Charles DiSogra, in *Diet, Nutrition, and Cancer Prevention: A Guide to Food Choices*, Public Health Service, National Institutes of Health Publication, no. 85-2711 (Washington, D.C., November 1984), pp. 32–41, and Oliver Alabaster, *The Power of Prevention* (New York: Simon and Schuster, 1986), pp. 281–291.
7. Ornish, pp. 46–47.

Chapter 12

1. Most current dietary guidelines recommended by major health-education organizations call for a daily intake of around 2,000 calories for the nonobese adult. To accomplish this, these guidelines suggest reducing or avoiding consumption of sugar, particularly in the form of commercially prepared baked goods and desserts. The 1986 American Heart Association Diet states that desserts and sweets high in sugar "are high in calories and low in nutritional value." For more details, see American Heart Association, *The American Heart Association Diet: An Eating Plan for Healthy Americans* (AHA National Center, 7320 Greenville Avenue, Dallas, TX 75231); World Health Organization, Expert Committee on Cardiovascular Desease, *Prevention of Coronary Heart Disease*, WHO Technical Report Series, no. 678 (Geneva, 1982), p. 23; and U.S. Department of Health and Human Services, "Diet, Nutrition and Cancer Prevention: A Guide to Food Choices," NIH Publication no. 85-2711 (November 1984), pp. 26, 28, 30.

2. Jane Brody, *Jane Brody's Good Food Book: Living the High-Carbohydrate Way* (New York: Norton, 1985), pp. 92–106.

3. J. W. Anderson *et al.*, "Hypocholesterolemic Effects of Oat-Bran or Bean Intake for Hypercholesterolemic Men," *American Journal of Clinical Nutrition* 40 (1984): 1152–1155.

4. Theresa Mondeika, "Cholesterol Content of Shellfish," *Journal of the American Medical Association* 254 (November 22–29, 1985): 2970.

5. Dr. Jan Stjernsward, interviewed by the authors (Geneva: World Health Organization, December 30, 1985).

Index